ELECTRON MICROSCOPIC ATLAS OF BRAIN TUMORS

ELECTRON MICROSCOPIC ATLAS OF BRAIN TUMORS

Tung Pui Poon, M.D.

Chief Neuropathologist, New York Medical College —
Metropolitan Hospital Center,
and Assistant Professor of Pathology,
New York Medical College, New York

Asao Hirano, M.D.

Head, Division of Neuropathology,
Montefiore Hospital and Medical Center,
and Professor of Pathology (Neuropathology),
Albert Einstein College of Medicine, New York

H. M. Zimmerman, M.D.

Chief, Department of Pathology,
Montefiore Hospital and Medical Center,
and Professor of Pathology,
Albert Einstein College of Medicine, New York

GRUNE & STRATTON
New York and London

Grune & Stratton, Inc.,
111 Fifth Avenue, New York, New York 10003

Library of Congress Catalog Card Number 70-175094
International Standard Book Number 0-8089-0740-9
Printed in the United States of America

CONTENTS

PREFACE

Many unsolved problems regarding the cytogenesis of some brain tumors face the student who employs conventional light microscopy as his major tool in diagnosis. A few examples may be cited: What is the cell of origin of the so-called gigantocellular neoplasm—is the tumor a glioma or a sarcoma? Is there a tumor in the cerebellum that is of mesodermal origin —a cerebellar sarcoma—and is this tumor different from the so-called medulloblastoma? What is the cell of origin of the acoustic neurilemoma? Similarly, what is the nature or cytogenesis of the cerebellar hemangioblastoma? Also, what are the tumors that are confined to the nervous system and have all the earmarks of extracranial malignant lymphomas?

These and similar questions concerning the origin of tumors of the nervous system can often be determined by high resolution microscopy, made possible by the electron microscope. This was one major consideration that prompted the preparation of this atlas. Another was the elucidation of the fine cellular structures that have engaged the interest of morphologists and cell biologists since the advent of the compound microscope. The ultramicroscopic appearance and often the functional significance of certain cytoplasmic organelles are of abiding interest. Of no less value is an understanding of neural neoplasia to an appreciation of the relationship of tumor cells to basement membrane structures, extracellular spaces, and blood vessel walls.

A considerable literature is in process of development on this subject, but as yet no inclusive publication is available. A list of pertinent references, by no means exhaustive, that should be of help to the investigator who desires to supplement the information contained in this volume is presented at the end of it. Citations are arranged according to subject matter and are not confined to tumor categories; the list also includes articles of a general nature that are of value in elucidating structures common to all cells, neoplastic and nonneoplastic.

Study of the various tumors illustrated will disclose the fact that most, but not all, gliomas are included. In addition, the meningiomas and neurilemomas are treated fairly comprehensively. Also portrayed are a number of other nongliomatous neoplasms. This atlas, however, cannot be considered definitive. The very nature of the technique involved in the preparation of the electron micrographs and the infrequent availability of some of the rarer tumors at operation preclude this. A long time will be needed for the supplementation of this work with the less frequently encountered neoplasms.

Two examples of metastatic tumors in the brain are included, first, because such lesions are encountered on occasion at operation without suspicion of their exact nature, and second, because their distinctive characteristics under the electron microscope are as easily recognizable as with light microscopy. Moreover, the relationship of the metastatic epithelial tumor cells to the extracellular spaces can hardly be appreciated in conventional photomicrographs. For somewhat similar reasons, a nonneoplastic space-occupying lesion in the brain, a chronic granuloma of cryptococcal origin, is included.

Perhaps some appreciation of the value of electron microscopy in the study of brain tumors of doubtful origin is afforded by the illustrations of the spinal epithelial cyst (Fig. 33 and Plates 60 and 61). The problem posed as to the nature of this cystic tumor under the light microscope, namely, whether it is a tumor of ependymal origin, is resolved in a manner unattainable without electron microscopy.

NOTES ON TECHNIQUE

Biopsy specimens of each tumor were obtained at the operating room table. Immediately after excision, parts of the specimen were taken for electron microscopic study while the rest was placed in 10% Formalin and then processed for conventional light microscopy. The specimens reserved for electron microscopic examination were cut into small blocks about 1 mm in diameter, and immersed in 5% glutaraldehyde in 1/15 M phosphate buffer, pH 7.4. Postfixation was in Dalton's chrome osmium for about 1 hour. After dehydration in an ascending series of alcohols and two changes of propylene oxide, the blocks were embedded in Epon. Thin sections were cut with a diamond knife and stained in uranyl and lead salts prior to examination in a Siemens 1A or RCA 3F electron microscope.

ABBREVIATIONS EMPLOYED
IN ILLUSTRATIONS

AsP	Astrocytic process
BM	Basement membrane
C	Cilia
Cen	Centriole
CG	Cytoplasmic granules
Chr	Chromatin
Col	Collagen
D	Dense body
Des	Desmosome
End	Endothelium
ER	Granular endoplasmic reticulum
ES	Extracellular space
f	Filaments (fibrils)
G	Golgi apparatus
Gly	Glycogen
IB	Inclusion body
L	Lumen
Li	Lipofuscin
Ly	Lysosome
M	Mitochondrion
MT	Microtubles
Mv	Microvilli
ncl	Nucleolus
NP	Nuclear pole
Nuc	Nucleus
Pl	Platelet
Pr	Cell process
RBC	Erythrocyte
RL	Rootlet
SG	Secretory granule
TF	Tonofilaments
V	Vesicle

ELECTRON MICROSCOPIC
ATLAS OF BRAIN TUMORS

ASTROCYTOMA

Under conventional light microscopy this neoplasm (*Fig. 1*) consists of large protoplasmic and smaller fibrillary astrocytes in a compact fibroglial stroma. Microcysts have coalesced to form larger cavities, and these in turn have fused into macrocysts (*at top of photomicrograph*). Hematoxylin-eosin stain; mag. x170.

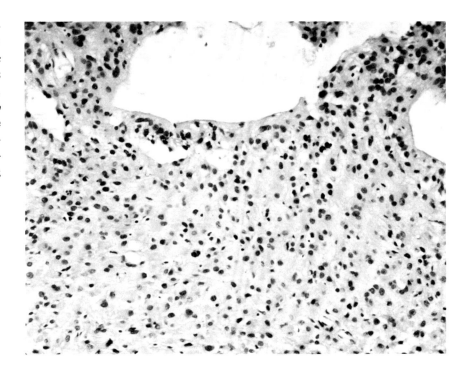

Plate 1. This electron micrograph reveals portions of several tumor cells of an astrocytoma. The nucleus is fairly regular in shape, and the chromatin is evenly distributed. The nucleolus is not present in this plane of section. The most conspicuous feature of the cytoplasm is the abundant glial fibrils (f). In addition, several microtubules (MT), mitochondria (M), dense bodies (D), vesicles (V), scattered elements of the rough endoplasmic reticulum (ER), and ribosomes are seen. Intercellular adhesive devices (*arrows*) are present between adjacent tumor cells. The extracellular space is quite narrow.

The cells comprising the astrocytoma are, in general, very similar morphologically to nonneoplastic reactive astrocytes.

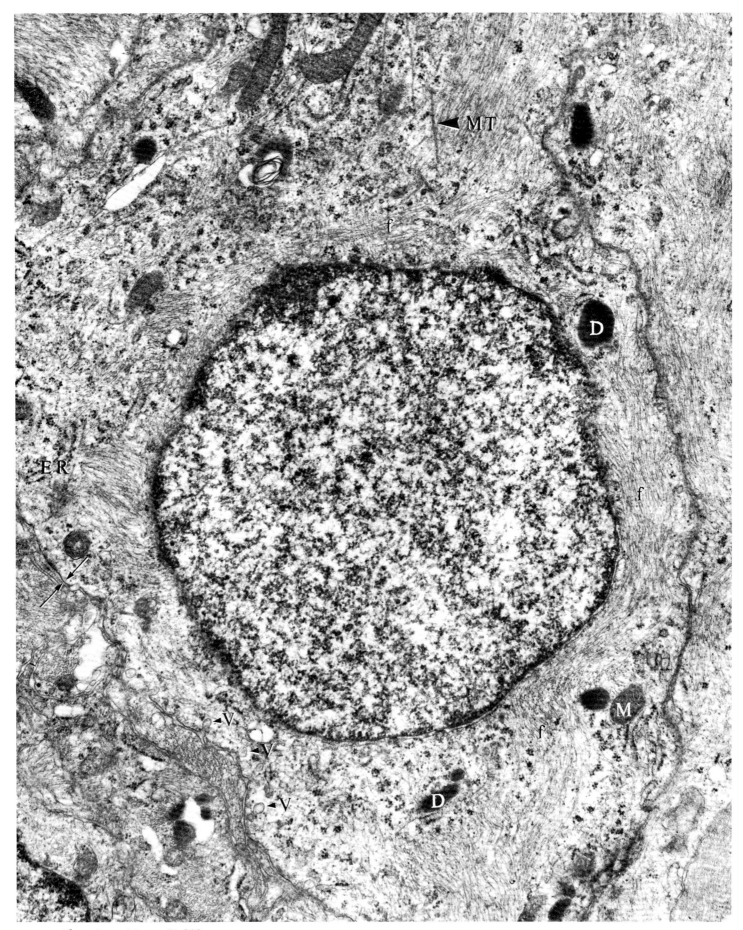

Plate 1   Mag. x19,000

3

Plate 2.   An electron micrograph of a common type of blood vessel found within astrocytomas. The basement membrane (BM) is completely invested by astrocytic foot processes (AsP). These contain variable numbers of glycogen granules (Gly). One side of the vascular lumen is lined by endothelial cells (End) containing a nucleus (Nuc) and mitochondria (M).

The relationship between the astrocytic foot processes and the blood vessel wall is identical to that observed in normal cerebral tissue. In the astrocytoma, however, astrocytic cells alone are present in addition to the blood vessels. Myelin and neuronal processes, including synapses, are generally excluded from the interior of the tumor mass although they may be present at its margins. The peripheral infiltration of the tumor cells accounts for the diversity of cell types, including neurons and normal glia, seen at the margins of astrocytomas.

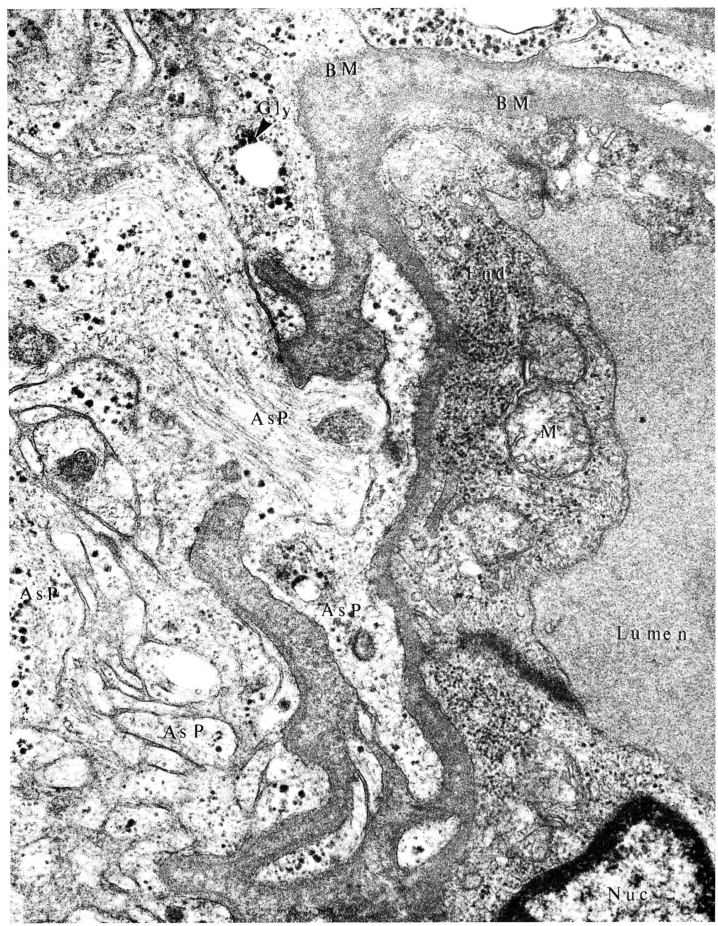

Plate 2   Mag. x50,000

5

Plate 3. Many blood vessels found within astrocytomas are surrounded by astrocytic foot processes which completely invest them as in normal brain. In this micrograph, however, the blood vessel is surrounded by wide extracellular spaces (ES). A prominent basement membrane (BM) is present which shows extensive infolding. Several nearby cell processes are completely surrounded by the basement membrane, external to which there are interspersed bundles of collagen fibers (Col). Note the similarity between the contents, other than erythrocytes (RBC), within the vascular lumen lined by endothelium (End) and the extracellular spaces (ES). This suggests edema of hematogenous origin. The large extracellular spaces probably result ultimately in the "microcysts" commonly observed with optical microscopy in certain astrocytomas (Fig. 1).

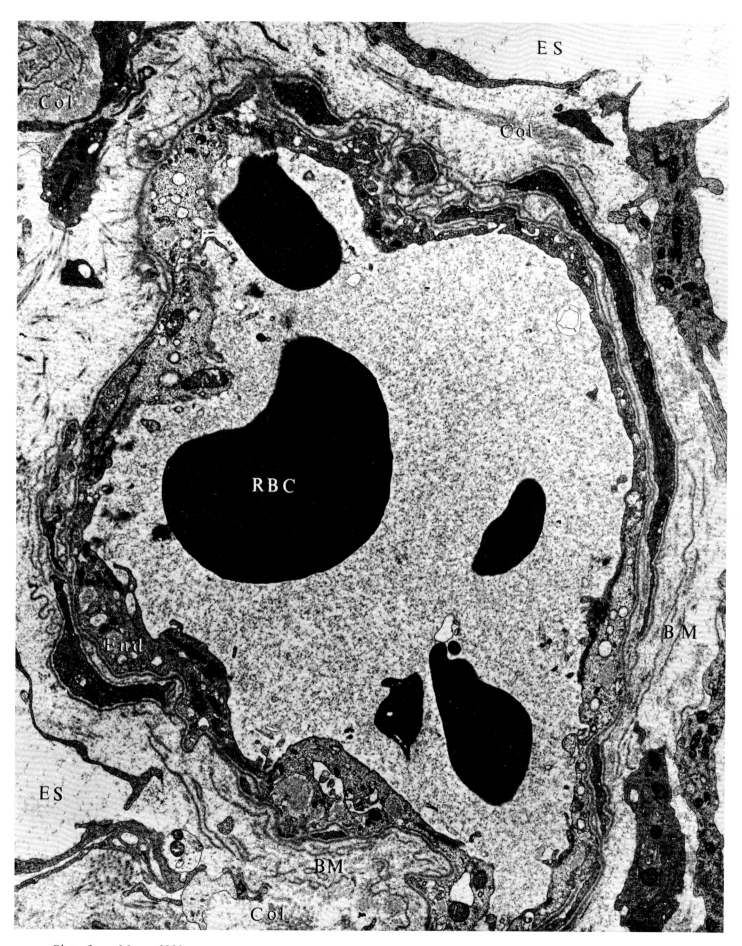

Plate 3   Mag. x6000

7

8

Fig. 2. Photomicrograph of a rapidly growing astrocytoma. Most of the tumor cells are readily identifiable as fibrillary and protoplasmic astrocytes. The fibroglial stroma is conspicuous, as are the several blood vessels in this illustration. A number of tumor cells, however, have large hyperchromatic nuclei of bizarre shape. It is these pleomorphic cells that suggest a "malignant" astrocytoma. Hematoxylin-eosin stain; mag. x325.

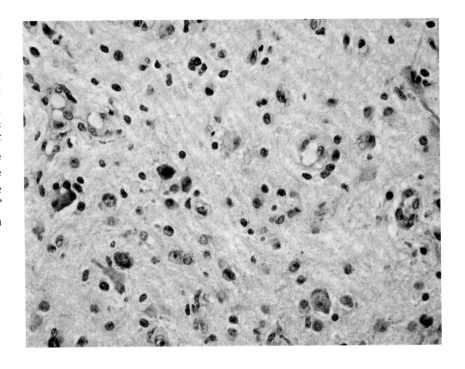

Plate 4. Part of a neoplastic astrocyte in a rapidly growing tumor. The nucleus (Nuc) has a rather irregular shape and a patchy distribution of its chromatin. Large extranuclear bundles of fibrils (f) are prominent, and occasional mitochondria (M) can be identified. In addition, several membrane-bounded dense-core vesicles, 500-800 Å in diameter, may be seen in the cytoplasm (*arrows*). Similar vesicles have been noted in reactive astrocytes in a case of subacute sclerosing leukoencephalitis.

In general, irregularity in size and shape of nuclei and cytoplasm seen in electron micrographs can be correlated with the degree of malignancy of glial tumors.

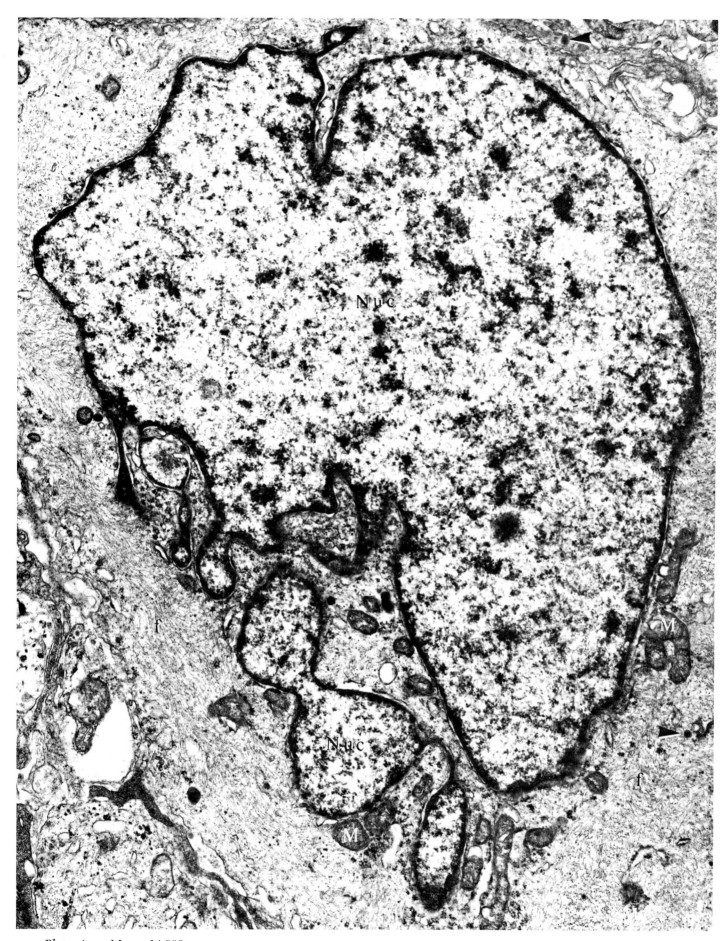

Plate 4   Mag. x14,000

9

Plate 5. *top:* Electron micrograph of a somewhat necrotic area in a glioma. Dense fibrillar bundles composed of glial filaments (f) are visible and are apparently resistant to necrotic disintegration. Cell membranes and other organelles are difficult to distinguish. Some bundles of the glial filaments appear to be granular (*asterisks*), but this is probably because the bundles are sectioned in oblique or transverse planes.

bottom: Intracellular glial filaments (f) sectioned in longitudinal and transverse planes. They measure 60-80 Å in diameter and are similar to, but smaller than, the 100 Å filaments which are normal components of neurons. Glycogen granules (Gly) are found among the glial filaments.

The filaments are apparently identical to those observed in both normal and reactive astrocytes. In all cases, at high resolution, they may be seen to contain electron-lucent centers, producing the appearance of hollow tubes. Within the central nervous system these filaments are generally characteristic of astrocytes, but they may be found in ependymal cells and, under certain conditions, also in reactive oligodendroglia.

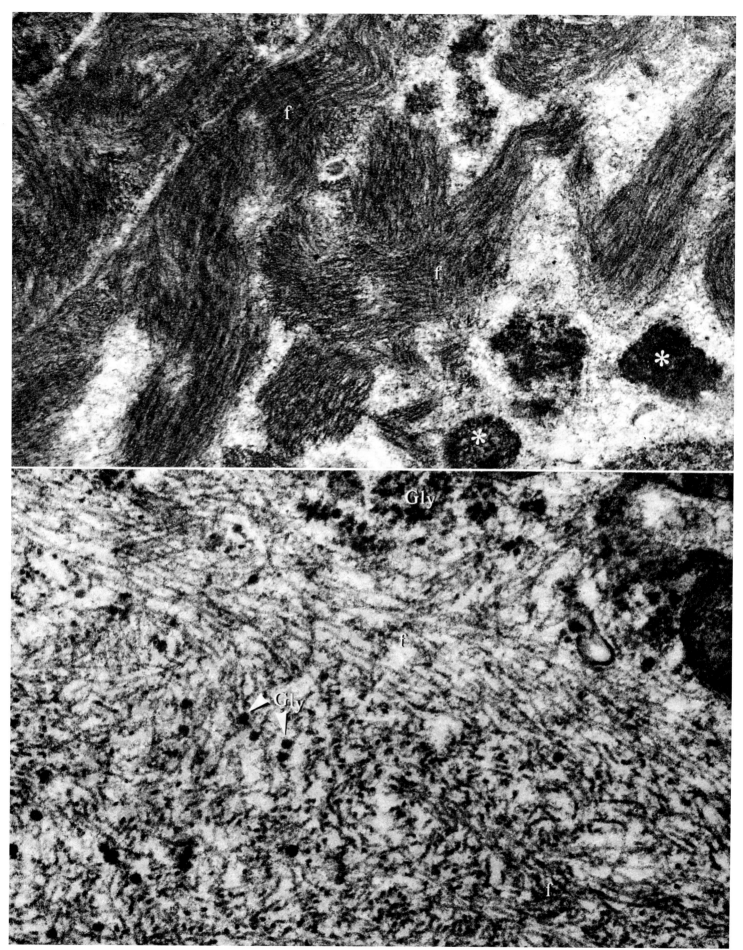

Plate 5   (*top*) Mag. x80,000.   (*bottom*) Mag. x100,000

11

GLIOBLASTOMA MULTIFORME

Pleomorphic cells of this neoplasm are arranged around some blood vessels and form pseudopalisades around central zones of necrosis (*Fig. 3*). The nuclei are often hyperchromatic and bizarre in shape; some cells are multinucleated. Hematoxylin-eosin stain; mag. x170.

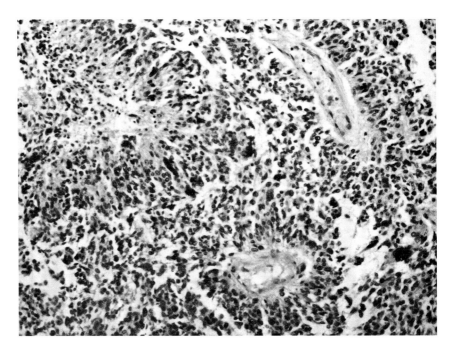

Pseudopalisading of spongioblasts are a prominent feature of this glioblastoma multiforme (*Fig. 4*). The spindle-shaped tumor cells lie in rows on the margins of acellular necrotic foci. Hematoxylin-eosin stain; mag. x130.

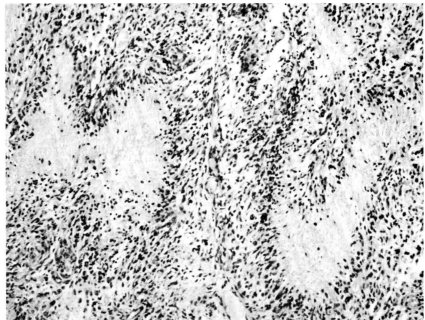

Plate 6. The cell in the center of the micrograph has relatively electron-lucent cytoplasmic ground substance. Scattered mitochondria (M) and elements of the rough endoplasmic reticulum are present. A Golgi apparatus (G) is also present, as are scattered ribosomes. The relatively clear cytoplasm is virtually filled with barely discernible, but definite, glial fibrils. Half desmosomes, facing a basement membrane-lined extracellular space, are seen at the arrows. A larger, collagen-containing (Col) extracellular space may be seen in the lower right-hand corner of the micrograph. Several cell processes contain less dense (1), denser (2), and much denser (3) cytoplasmic matrices that surround the tumor cell whose nucleolus (ncl) is quite irregular in shape. The least dense cell process (1) contains few or no glial fibrils, while some of the denser processes (2) contain more fibrils than the cell in the center of the micrograph.

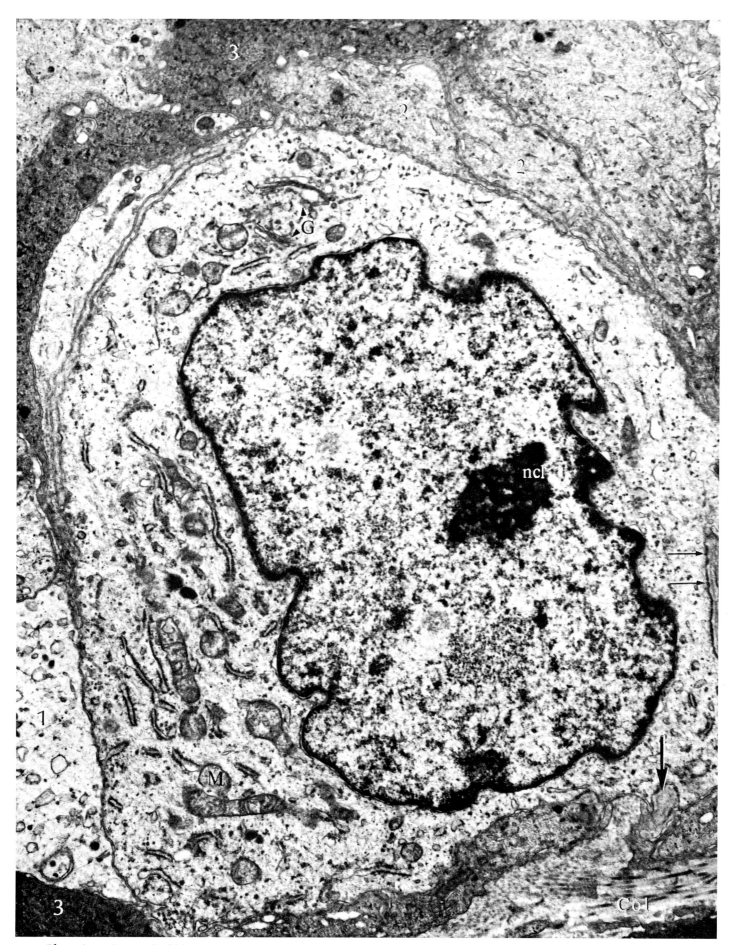

Plate 6   Mag. x31,000

13

Photomicrograph (*Fig.* 5) of multinucleated giant cells in glioblastoma multiforme. Hematoxylin-eosin stain; mag. x250.

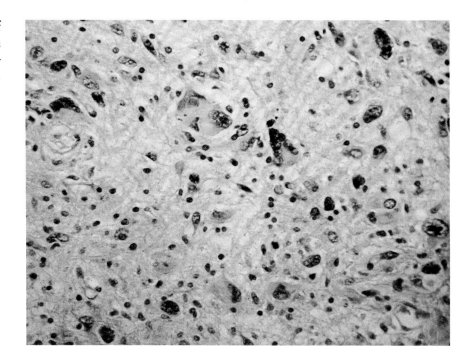

Plate 7. The large cell in the center of the micrograph contains five sections of nuclei (Nuc), two with nucleoli (ncl). The cytoplasm is fairly dense due to the presence of abundant, fine glial fibrils (f). Numbers of mitochondria (M) are also present. Short cell processes protrude into the large, relatively clear, extracellular spaces (ES), which contain some collagen (Col). The arrowheads point to the cytoplasmic cell membrane which delimits the tumor cell in the center of the micrograph. A degenerating cell is visible in the lower right-hand corner.

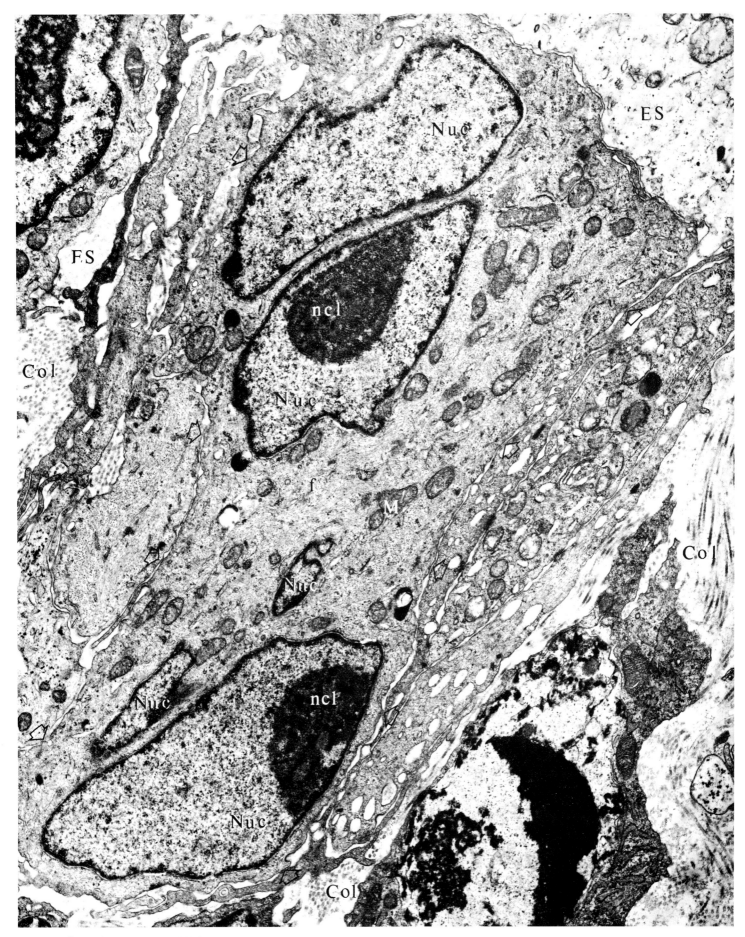

Plate 7   Mag. x25,000

15

Plate 8. The tumor cell in the center of this electron micrograph contains numerous mitochondria, glial fibrils (f), ribosomes, and cisternae of the rough endoplasmic reticulum (ER), resulting in a dense, crowded appearance of the cytoplasm. The cell surface is extensively folded, and the cell processes (Pr) of other, fibril-containing, cells interdigitate and protrude within the cytoplasm of the centrally situated tumor cell. The nucleus (Nuc) is extremely irregular in outline and has a bizarre appearance. Extracellular spaces (ES) are large and readily identifiable.

In keeping with the name of this malignant tumor, the cells display a great variety of cell densities, shapes, sizes, and contents.

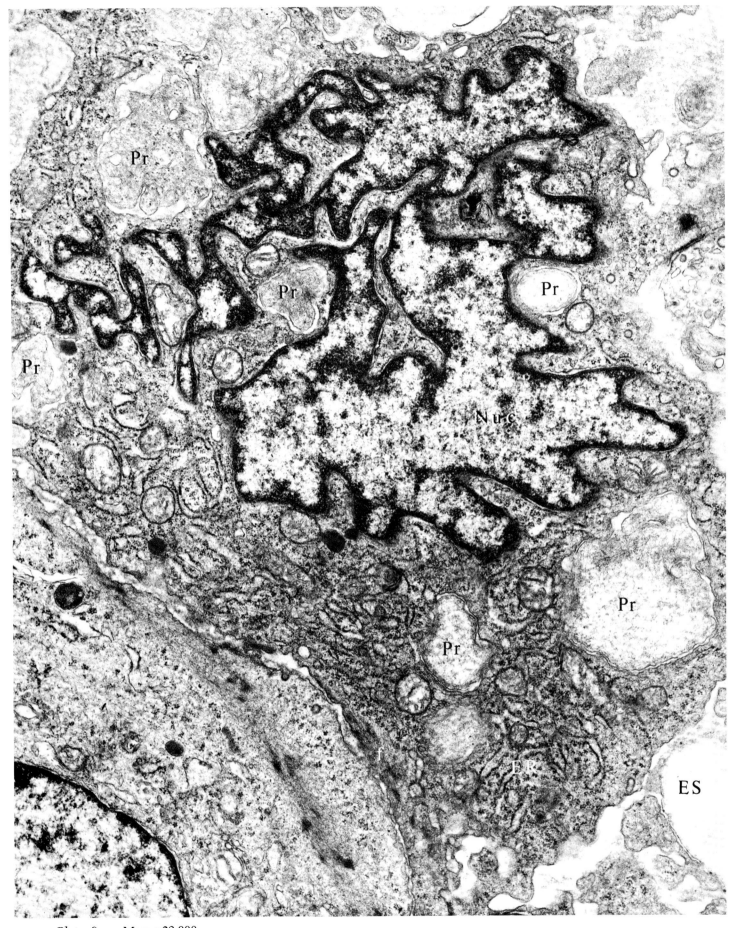

Plate 8   Mag. x23,000

17

Plate 9.   An apparently viable tumor cell is seen in a huge extracellular space (ES). The latter contains hematogenous edema fluid, scattered cell processes (Pr), and the remains of necrotic cells. The tumor cells in this micrograph are packed with glial fibrils (f). The nucleus (Nuc) in the cell in the upper half of the illustration is extensively infolded, and this has resulted in cytoplasmic invaginations within the nucleus. Such invaginations have sometimes been mistaken for intranuclear inclusions by light microscopy (see Fig. 19).

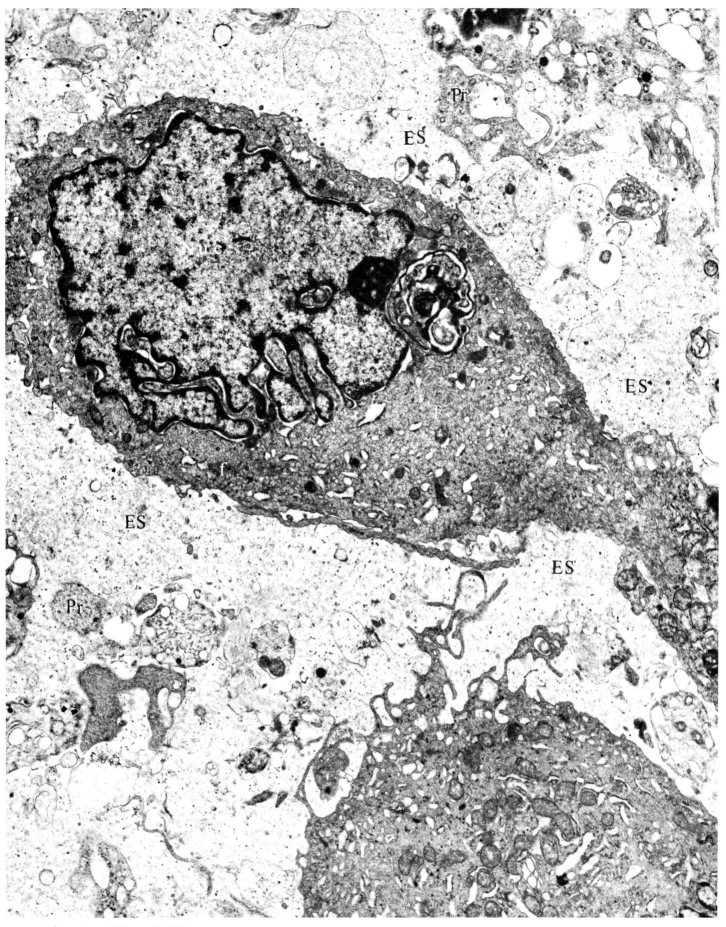

Plate 9   Mag. x25,000

Plate 10. The tumor cell in this micrograph has a large, well-preserved nucleus (Nuc) as well as glial fibrils (f) and mitochondria (M) in its cytoplasm. The large extracellular space (ES) which surrounds it is filled, in contrast to the previous illustration (Plate 9), with numerous collagen fibers (Col).

Although the central nervous system normally contains very little connective tissue, necrotic regions of tumor, especially glioblastoma multiforme, may contain abundant mesodermal elements. This is particularly pronounced around blood vessels within necrotic areas. At times the connective tissue proliferation is extensive enough to constitute a sarcoma that grows side by side with the malignant glioma.

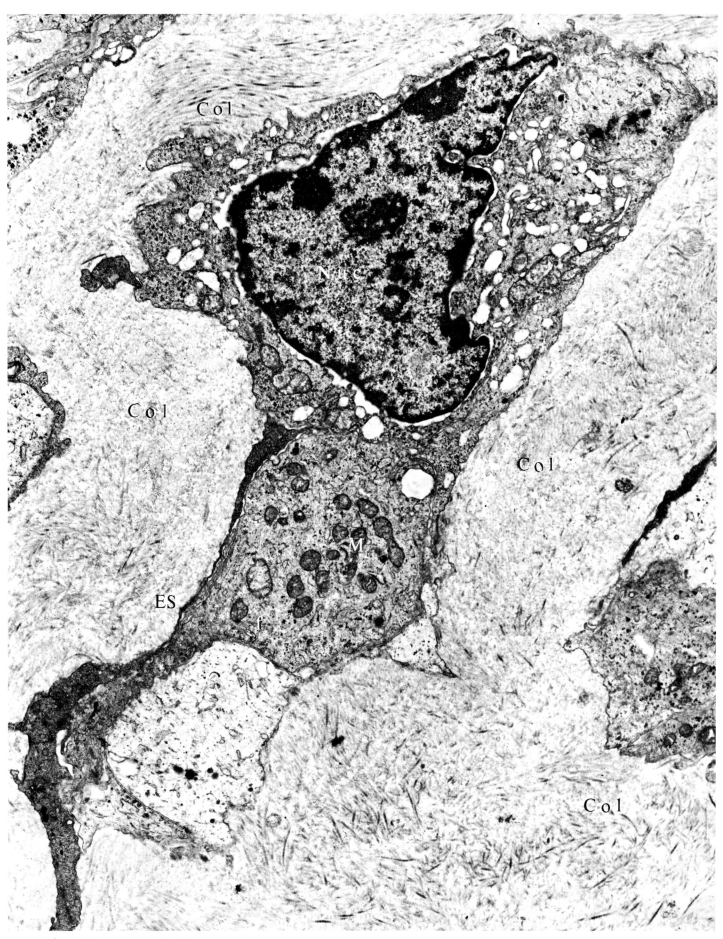

Plate 10　　Mag. x25,000

GIGANTOCELLULAR (MONSTROCELLULAR) GLIOBLASTOMA

Photomicrograph of a gigantocellular glioblastoma *(Fig. 6)* with large perivascular tumor cells and bizarre, multinucleated giant cells. Hematoxylin-eosin stain; mag. x300.

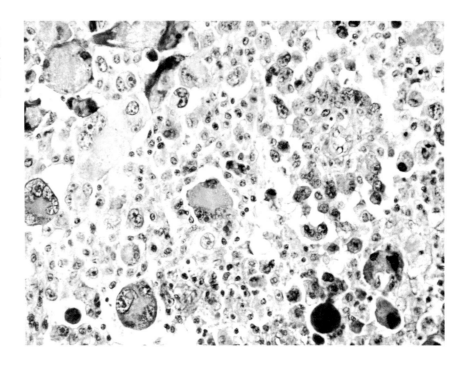

Plate 11. The tumor cell in the center of the micrograph contains several nuclear profiles (Nuc). One of these is surrounded by concentrically arranged glial filaments (f). Mitochondria (M), a Golgi apparatus (G), and ribosomes are present at the periphery of the cell. Prominent microtubules (MT) can also be seen in the cytoplasm. The cell membrane is indicated by arrowheads. Surrounding the cell, there are dense cell processes that contain considerably more rough endoplasmic reticulum. These cell processes in turn are surrounded by a wide extracellular space (ES) which contains collagen fibers (Col). Another tumor cell containing glial fibrils (f) may be seen in the lower portion of the micrograph.

The cellular origin of this type of neoplasm is the subject of some debate. Certain features of these tumors are suggestive of an astrocytic origin: the manner of cellular infiltration and invasion, the absence of collagen fibers in many areas, and the presence of glial fibrils as in the tumor cells of malignant astrocytomas.

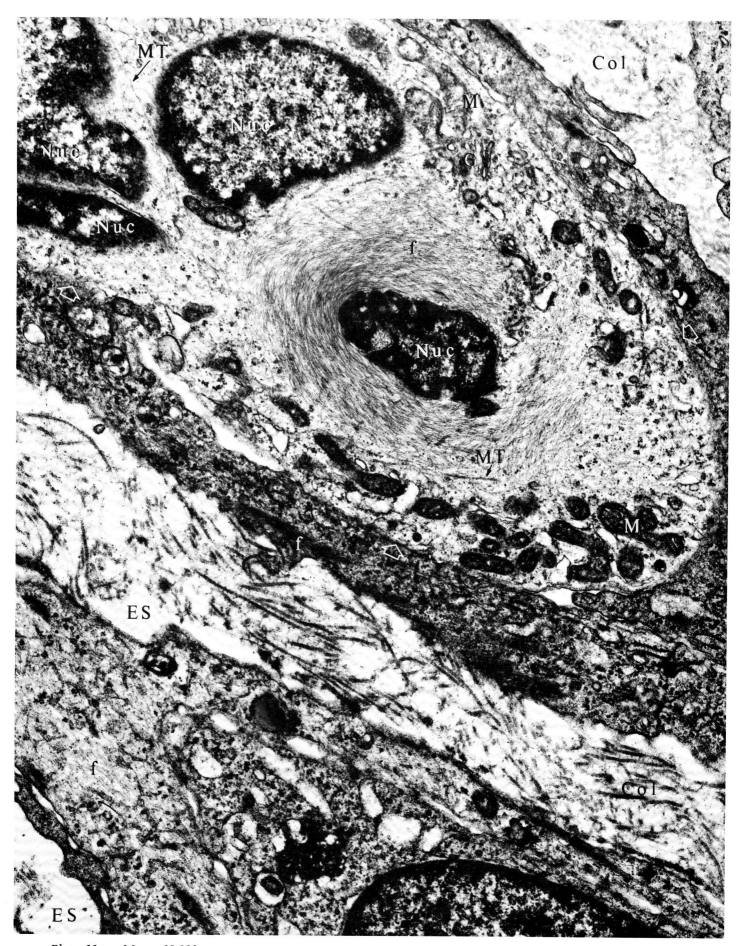

Plate 11   Mag. x28,000

23

Plate 12. The tumor cell in the lower right-hand corner of the micrograph has infiltrated an area of white matter containing myelinated axons. Arrowheads mark the edge of the tumor cell. A blood vessel lined by endothelium (End) and containing an erythrocyte (RBC) in its lumen is present in the upper half of the micrograph. A clearly defined basement membrane (BM) forms part of the vessel wall and coats the tumor cell on the surface exposed to the perivascular space. The nucleus of this cell is large and irregular in shape, and contains both a large and a small cytoplasmic invagination that have large numbers of fibrils (f). Nuclear pores around the cytoplasmic invaginations are marked by small white arrowheads. The remainder of the cellular cytoplasm also has many fibrils as well as mitochondria (M). Cell processes (Pr) and distended extracellular spaces (ES) are seen.

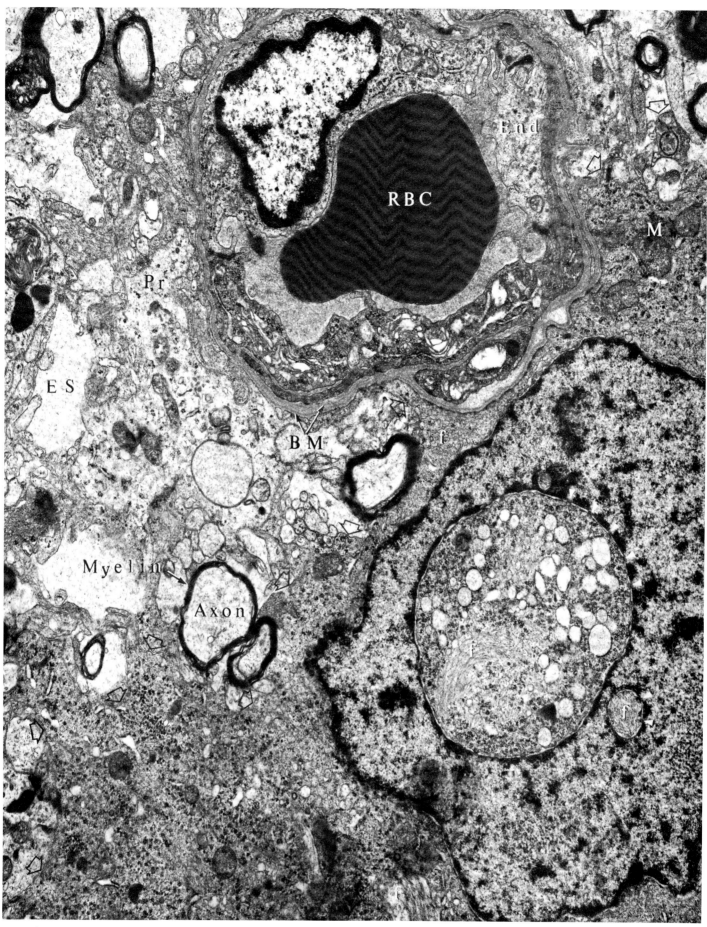

Plate 12   Mag. x30,000

Plate 13. Electron micrograph of several tumor cells whose cytoplasm is crowded with glial fibrils (f). Scattered mitochondria (M) and ribosomes are also present. The irregularities in the nuclear shapes have resulted in apparent intranuclear cytoplasmic inclusions. Two membrane-bounded dense-core vesicles, 500 Å in diameter, are present within encircled areas.

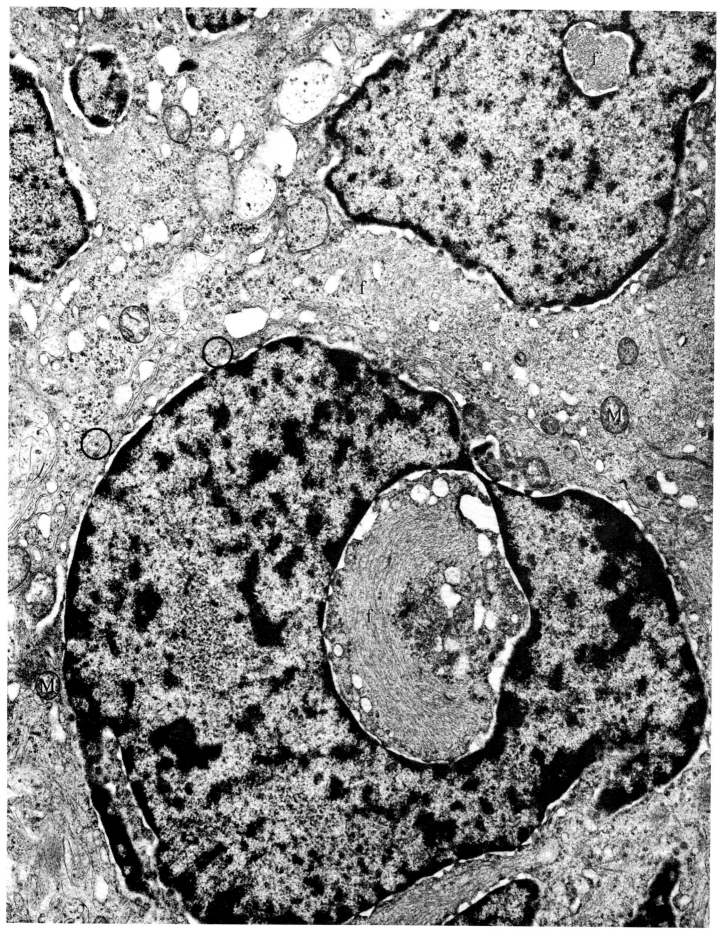

Plate 13   Mag. x28,000

27

Plate 14.   A tumor cell whose cytoplasm contains few, if any, glial fibrils. Mitochondria (M) and rough endoplasmic reticulum are present. The nucleus is irregular in shape and appears to be separated into two parts, one of which has the nucleolus (ncl). The cell is surrounded by a large extracellular space (ES).

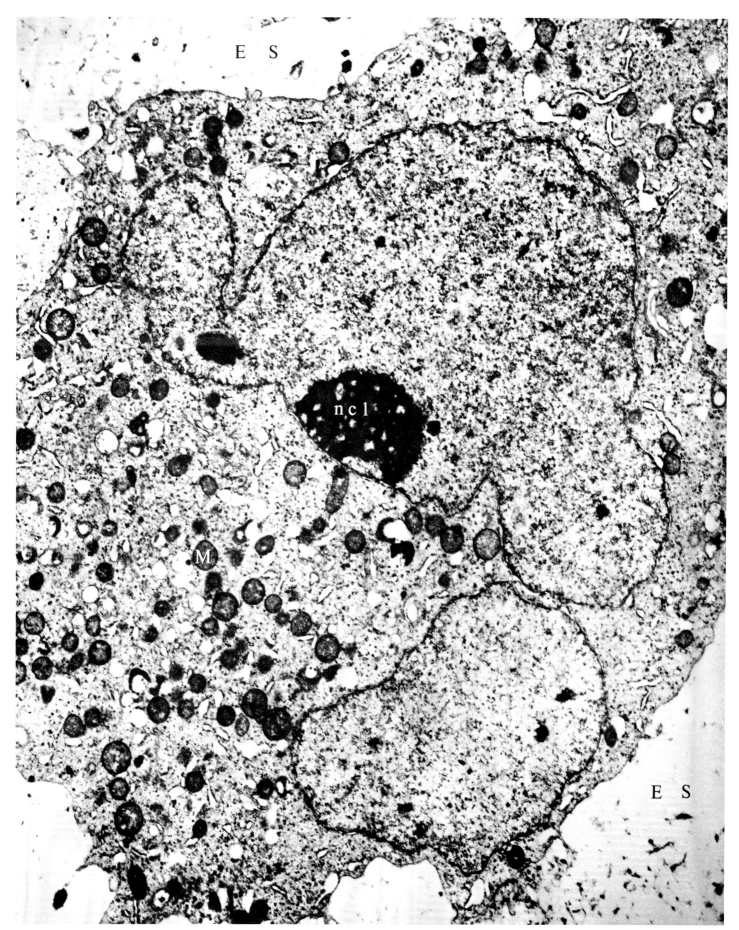

Plate 14   Mag. x14,000

EPENDYMOMA

Photomicrograph of an ependymoma of the fourth ventricle (*Fig. 7*). The small, dark, undifferentiated cells are arranged in rosettes around blood vessels and around presumably empty spaces (at this magnification). Hematoxylin-eosin stain; mag. x170.

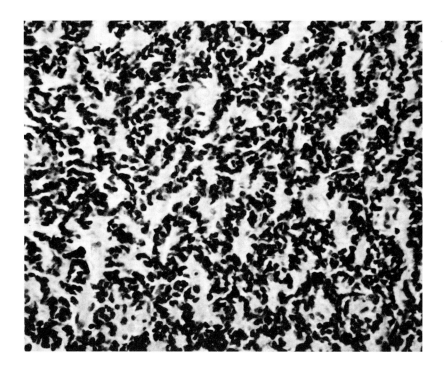

Plate 15. A nucleus of a tumor cell containing a prominent round nucleolus is present in the upper left-hand corner of the electron micrograph. The three main characteristics of the normal ependymal cell, namely, microvilli (Mv), cilia (C), and junctional apparatuses (*arrows*) are present in this neoplastic cell. The arrangement and order of these structures, however, are profoundly distorted. The cilia and microvilli, instead of extending into the ventricular lumen, are crowded together in a small extracellular space which is indented deep within the ependymal cytoplasm. Instead of the cellular monolayer found in normal ependyma, the tumor cells are arranged in a compact, solid mass so that junctional apparatuses, normally found only on the lateral edges, are irregular and are randomly distributed over the cell surface.

Similar arrangements of crowded cilia and microvilli have been reported in certain presumably normal laboratory animals. In these instances, however, the findings were relatively rare and the cells did not form a tumor mass.

The cytoplasm of the tumor cell in this micrograph contains microtubules (MT) and mitochondria (M). Adjacent cells have glial filaments (f).

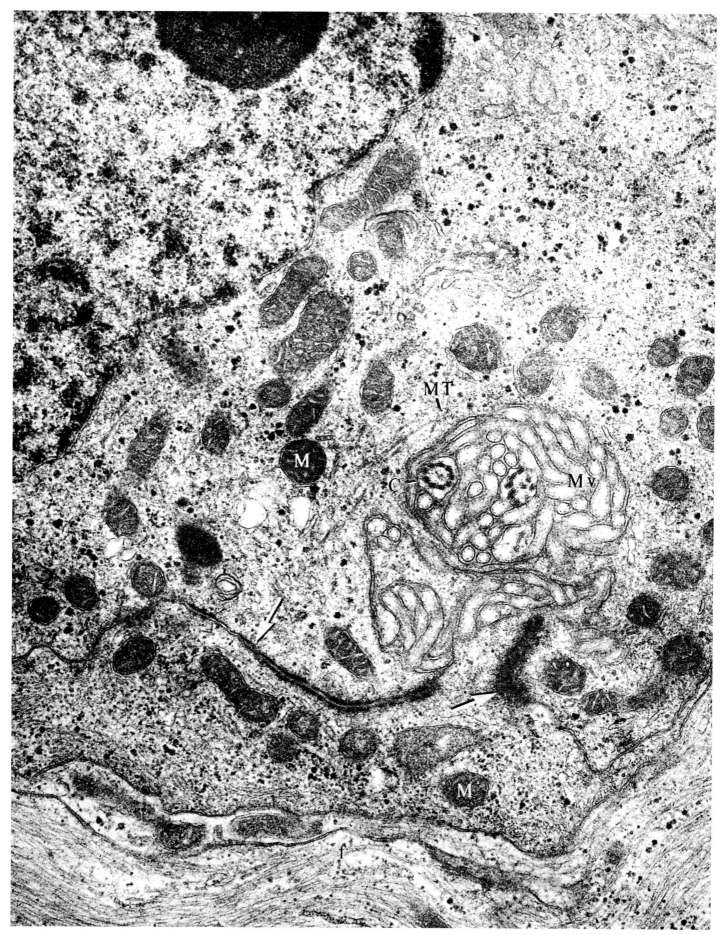

Plate 15   Mag. x40,000

31

Plate 16. Higher magnification of an area similar to that illustrated in the previous micrograph (Plate 15). Well-developed junctional complexes (*arrows*) are present between three adjacent tumor cells. At the left in the micrograph, tightly packed microvilli (Mv) are seen crowded into a diminutive extracellular space. Mitochondria (M) are present in the cytoplasm of the tumor cells.

The junctional complexes seen here are very similar to those found in normal ependyma. They differ somewhat, however, from the complexes seen in craniopharyngioma and metastatic carcinoma (Plates 44 and 55).

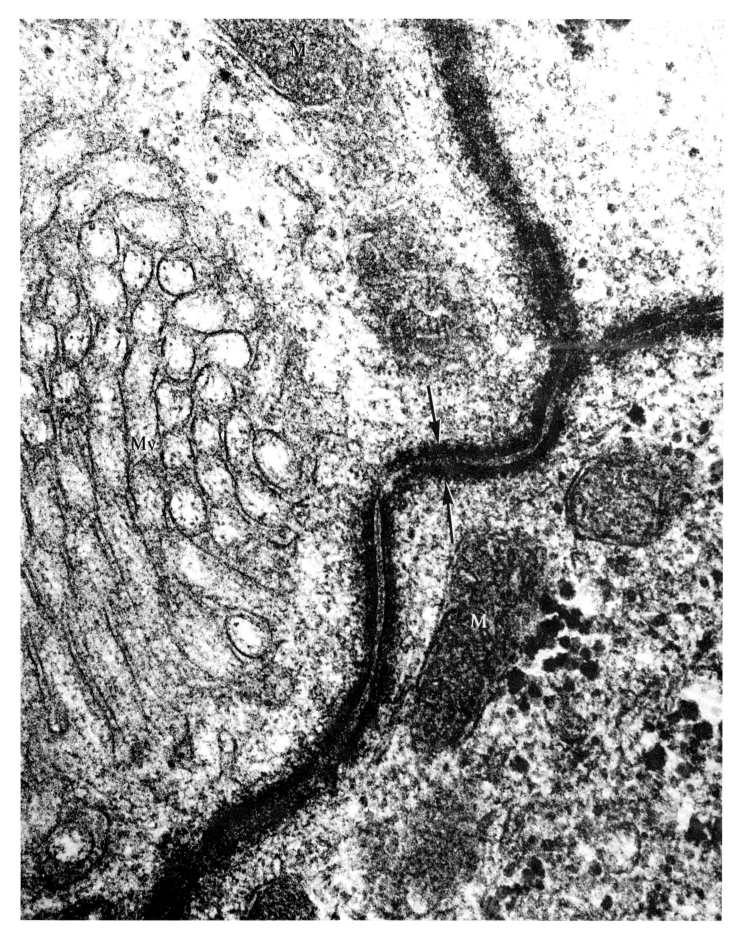

Plate 16   Mag. x96,000

33

Fig. 8. Photomicrograph of rosettes in an ependymoma. The pear-shaped tumor cells send fibrils towards the vascular adventitiae. Phosphotungstic acid-hematoxylin stain; mag. x350.

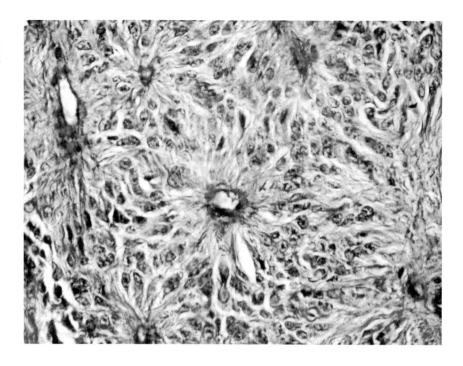

Plate 17. This is a low-magnification micrograph of a rosette, one of the characteristic features of ependymoma. A blood vessel lumen is visible at the upper margin of the illustration and is lined by endothelium (End). The perinuclear areas of numerous tumor cells are visible in the lower half of the picture. The nuclei (Nuc) are surrounded by narrow rims of cytoplasm, and delicate cell processes extend from the perinuclear areas towards the blood vessel. The perivascular area is crowded with many cell processes.

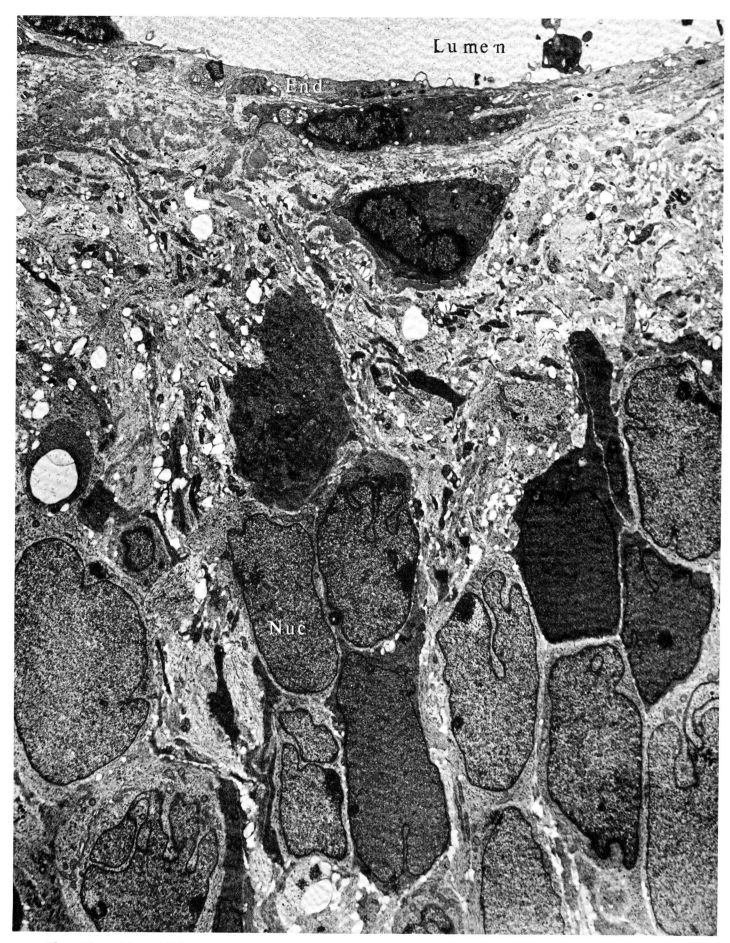

Lumen

End

Nuc

Plate 17   Mag. x6000.

35

Plate 18.   Section of ependymoma in the region of a blood vessel whose lumen, lined by endothelial cells (End), is visible at the upper margin of the micrograph. Portions of tumor cell nuclei (Nuc) are present in the lower right corner. Between the tumor cell nuclei and the vascular endothelium there are numerous cell processes (Pr) as well as fairly large extracellular spaces (ES) infiltrated with material similar to that found within the vascular lumen. Three platelets (Pl) are visible at the luminal surface of the endothelium. Two of the platelets show pronounced pseudopod formation. This configuration may be related to an early stage of thrombus formation.

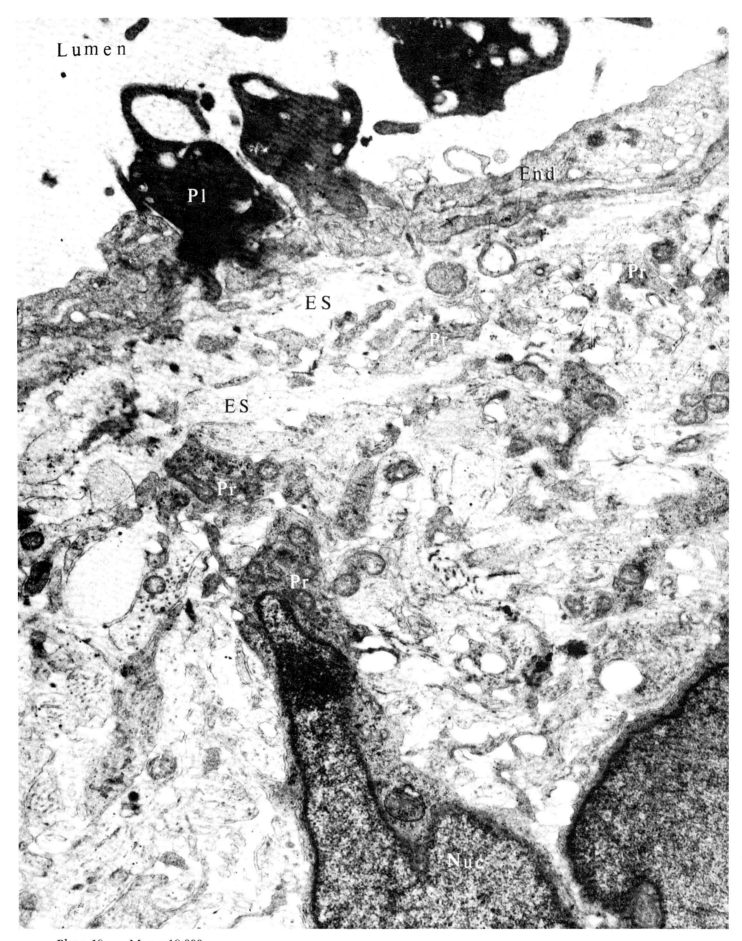

Lumen

Pl

ES

ES

Pr

Pr

End

Pr

Pr

Nuc

Plate 18   Mag. x18,000

37

Plate 19. top: In contrast to previously described ependymomas, others, such as the one illustrated here, show no cilia, microvilli, or junctional complexes. The tumor cells are closely packed. In addition to the usual organelles such as mitochondria (M), the cytoplasm contains microtubules (*arrowheads*).

bottom: The cytoplasm of the ependymoma cell contains numerous microtubules (MT). Both transverse (*arrows*) and longitudinal sections through the microtubules are visible. The dark structures in the lower portion of the micrograph are mitochondria (M). Microtubules are components of normal ependymal cells, but they are usually confined to the apical region of the cytoplasm and cilia. In tumor cells they are randomly distributed throughout the cells but are especially abundant in the processes.

Ependymal cells may sometimes contain glycogen granules and/or glial filaments. These, too, are normal constituents of ependymal cells. In reactive ependymal cells they are often more pronounced than in neoplastic cells. Surprisingly, secretory granules have been reported in ependymoma of the filum terminale of the spinal cord.

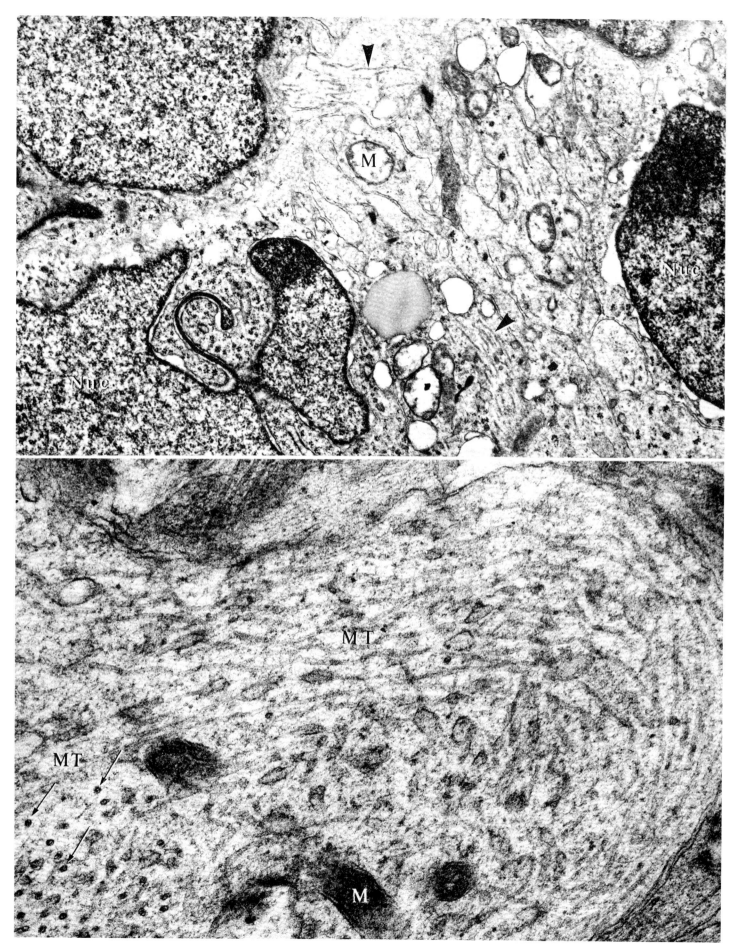

Plate 19   (*top*) Mag. x18,000.   (*bottom*) Mag. x80,000

EPENDYMOBLASTOMA

Fig. 9. Photomicrograph of an ependymoblastoma. The tumor cells are large, hyperchromatic, and form imperfect rosettes. Hematoxylin-eosin stain; mag. x375.

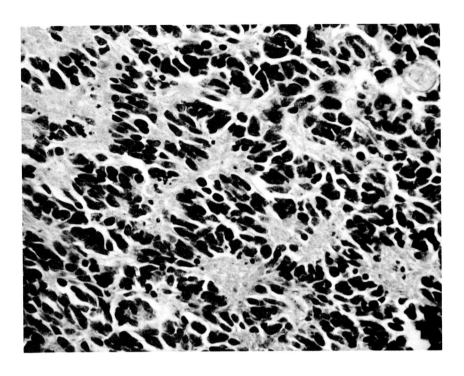

Plate 20. The tumor cells of this ependymoblastoma are closely packed. The nuclei show distinct margination of the chromatin (Chr) and have prominent nucleoli (ncl). No specializations of normal ependymal cytoplasm are present in the neoplastic cells, which contain the usual cytoplasmic organelles including granular endoplasmic reticulum (ER). The density of the cytoplasmic ground substance as well as the size and shape of the mitochondria (M) differ from cell to cell in this more malignant tumor.

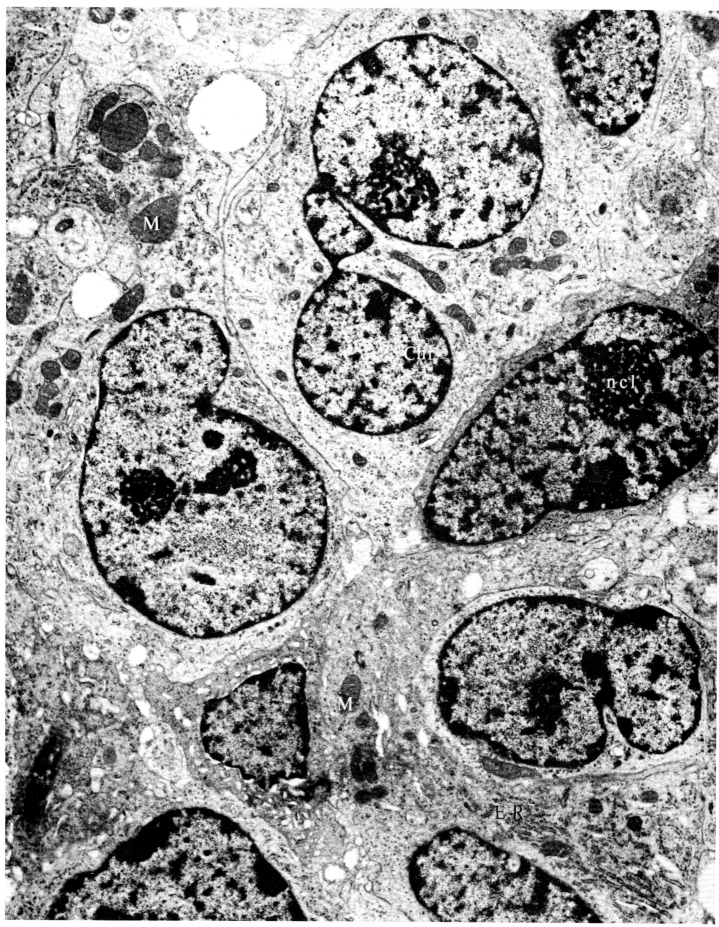

Plate 20   Mag. x8000

41

Fig. 10. Highly undifferentiated ependymoblastoma. The neoplastic cells are arranged in a poorly formed rosette around a blood vessel and send their apical processes to the vessel wall. Some cells are in mitotic division. Hematoxylin-eosin stain; mag. x375.

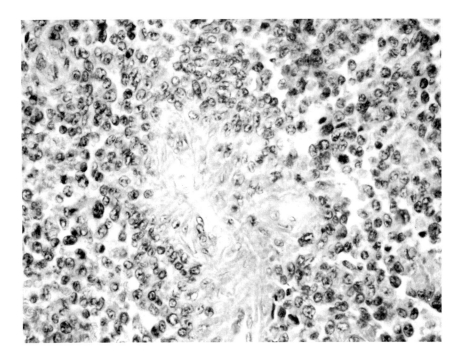

Plate 21. Section through a blood vessel in an ependymoblastoma. The plasma-filled lumen (L) of the vessel is lined by endothelial cells which are themselves surrounded by a distended extracellular space (ES) filled with several layers of basement membrane and infiltrated plasma. On the periphery of the perivascular region there are ependymoblastoma cells, some of which display half desmosomes (*arrowheads*) such as are present in normal ependyma which abuts on a perivascular space. Neither glial filaments nor microtubules are present in the tumor cells.

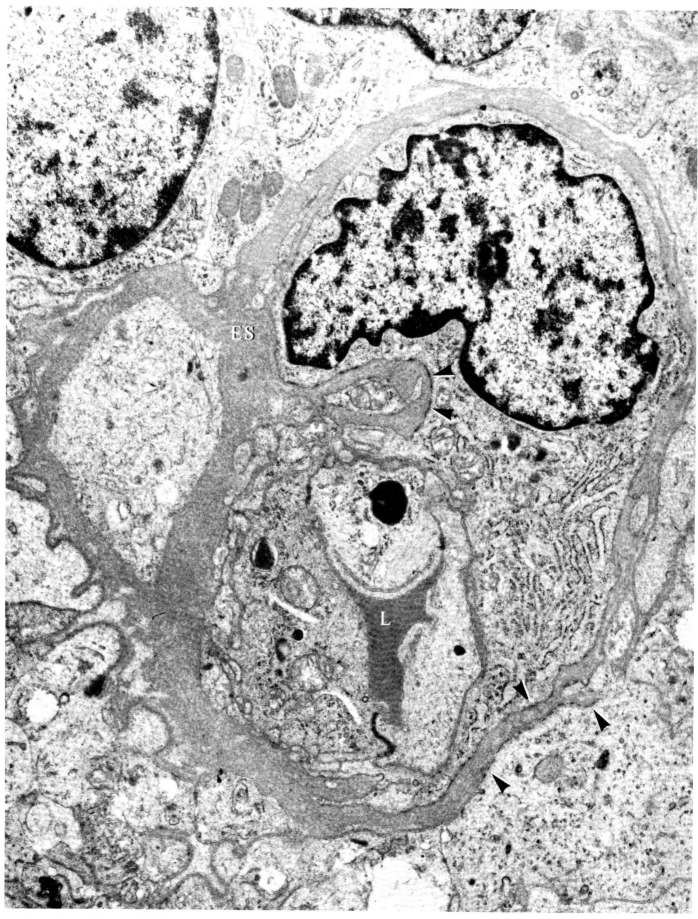

Plate 21   Mag. x17,000

OLIGODENDROGLIOMA

Fig. 11. Photomicrograph of a classical oligodendroglioma. The tumor presents a uniform picture with vascularized septa subdividing groups of cells into lobules. Each neoplastic cell has a round nucleus, and its clear cytoplasm produces an effect of a perinuclear halo. Hematoxylin-eosin stain; mag. x325.

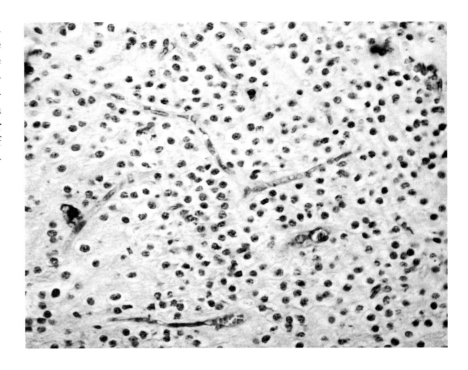

Plate 22. The uniform cells form a compact mass. The nuclei (Nuc) are spherical with homogeneously distributed chromatin. The cytoplasm also appears uniform and has no distinctive inclusions. Small extracellular spaces are crowded with narrow cell processes. In contrast to the usual appearance of the cells of an oligodendroglioma seen with the light microscope, no perinuclear haloes or large vacuoles are present. The cytoplasm contains mitochondria (M). There is no extensive extracellular space present, which seems to indicate that the haloes seen with light microscopy are the result of preparative artifact.

Others have reported abundant intercellular spaces in an oligodendroglioma that apparently accounted for the perinuclear haloes. Polygonal crystalline structures have also been reported in this tumor, but these are apparently rare and unusual features in gliomas.

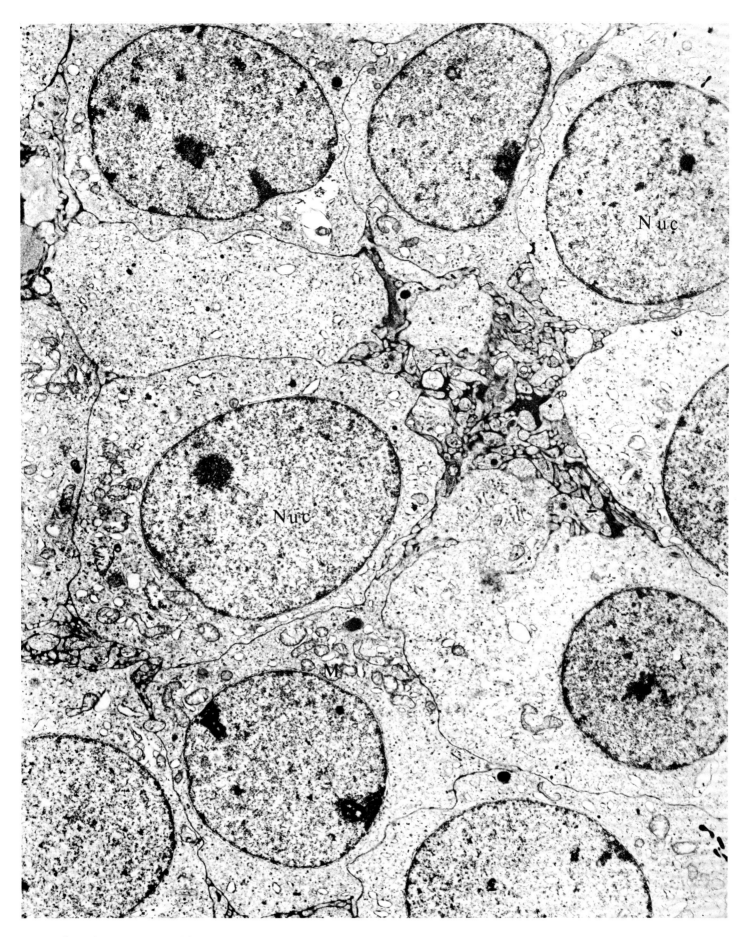

Plate 22   Mag. x8000

45

Plate 23. Higher magnification of a tumor cell similar to those illustrated in Plate 22. The cytoplasm contains mitochondria (M), dense bodies, ribosomes, and scattered vacuoles. Only few microtubules (MT) are present, but no glial filaments are seen. Junctional complexes are absent. The extracellular space is narrow but is distinct because of the presence of dense hematogenous edema fluid.

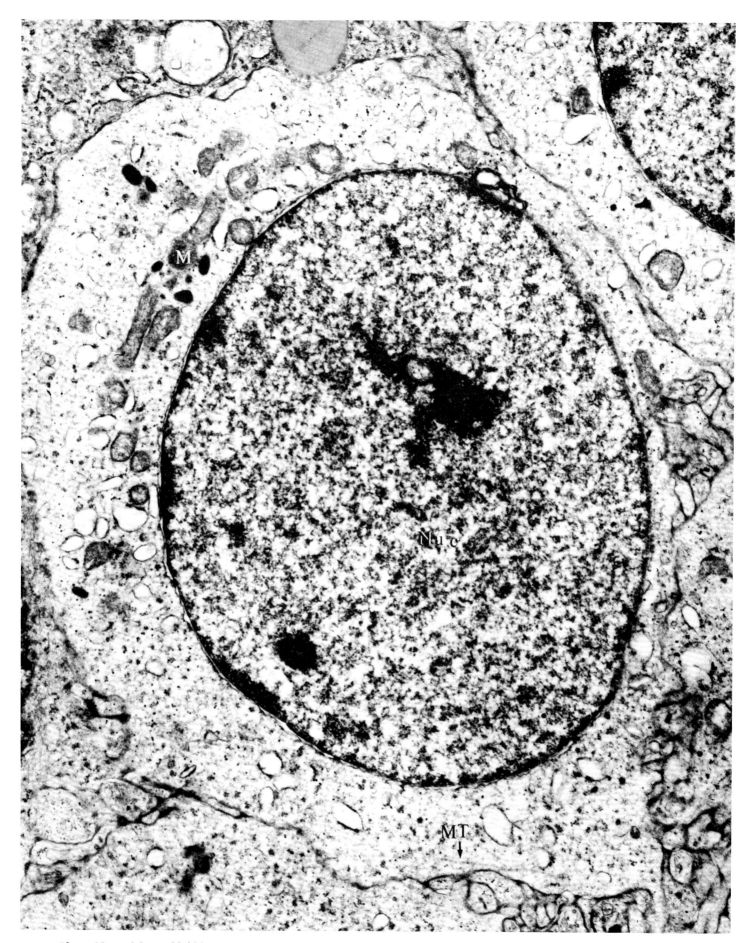

Plate 23   Mag. x38,000

Plate 24. This oligodendroglioma also contains astrocytic and ependymal cells. The cell (1) in the central portion of the micrograph resembles an oligodendrocyte. A granular inclusion body (IB), surrounded by a clear zone, is present in the nucleus (Nuc), which also contains two nucleoli (ncl) at opposite sides. Such inclusion bodies have been reported in a variety of both neoplastic and nonneoplastic cells.

The cell process (2), immediately below the central cell, contains prominent glial filaments (f) and is probably of astrocytic origin. It lies adjacent to the collagen-filled (Col) extracellular space (ES) and is coated by a narrow basement membrane.

At the top of the micrograph, a cell process (3) with dense cytoplasm can be seen that contains minute vesicles (V), microtubules, and glial filaments.

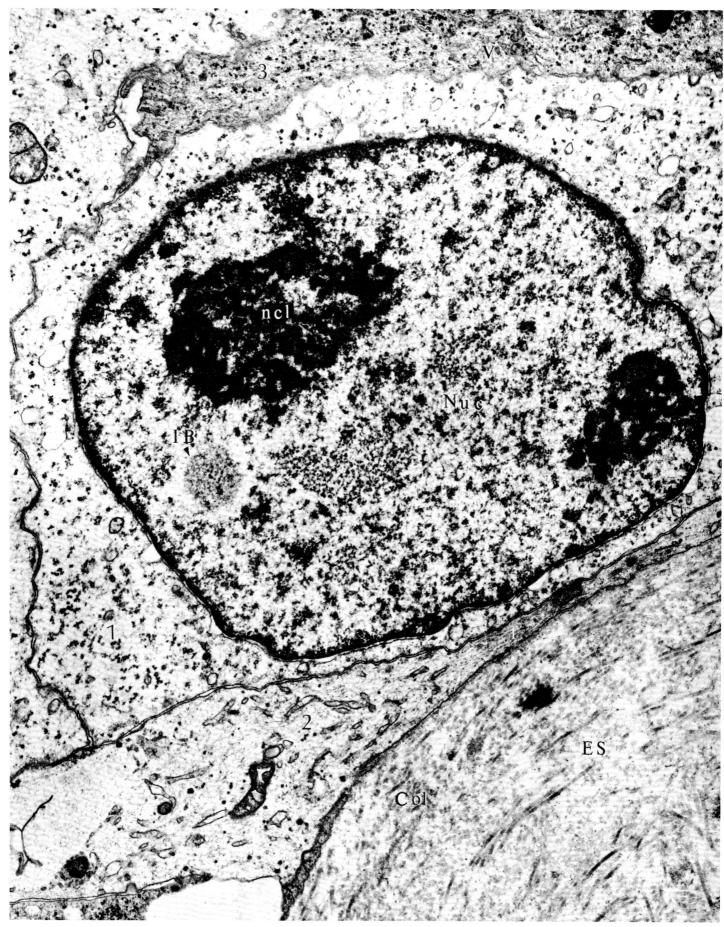

Plate 24   Mag. x38,000

MIXED GLIOMAS

EPENDYMOMA AND ASTROCYTOMA

Fig. 12. Photomicrograph of ependymomatous portion of a tumor composed in part of an ependymoma and in part of an astrocytoma. A rosette is present in the upper left corner of the illustration, and just to the right of center there is an acinar structure lined by ciliated columnar ependymal cells as seen in a medulloepithelioma. Hematoxylin-eosin stain; mag. x325.

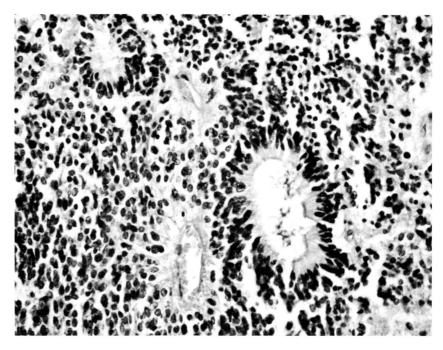

Fig. 13. This represents the astrocytoma portion of the same neoplasm illustrated in Fig. 12. These cells produce a stroma of glial fibrils. Hematoxylin-eosin stain; mag. x250.

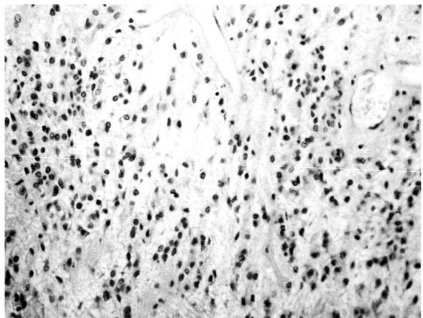

Plate 25. A ciliated tumor cell (C), derived from ependyma, is visible in the upper right-hand corner of the micrograph. A well-developed junctional complex, another characteristic of ependymal cells, is seen between the arrows. This cell also contains rootlets (RL) and mitochondria (M). On the left side of the illustration there is a section of a tumor cell through the perinuclear (Nuc) area that is filled with glial fibrils (f). Several cell processes in the field show similar fibrils. While reactive ependymal cells often contain many such fibrils, it is reasonable to assume that the fibril-containing cells in this illustration are astrocytes. This view is supported by the light microscopic appearance of the neoplasm.

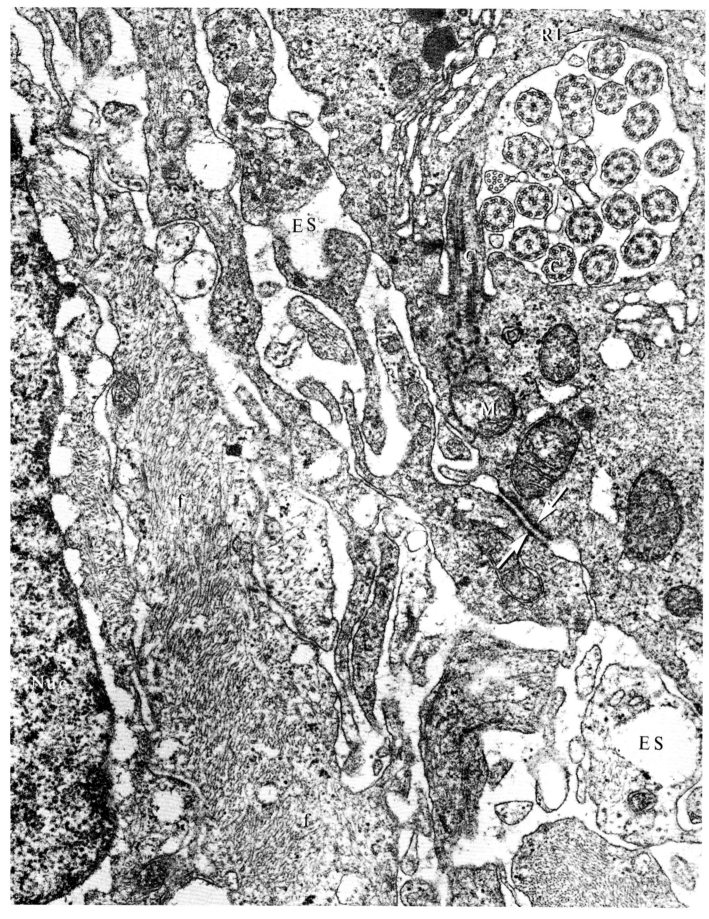

Plate 25   Mag. x49,000

EPENDYMOMA AND OLIGODENDROGLIOMA

Plate 26. This is a micrograph of an ependymomatous area of a mixed ependymoma and oligodendroglioma. Well-developed junctional complexes are visible (*small arrows*). Large aggregates of microvilli (*asterisks*), similar to those often seen in ependymomas, crowd a small extracellular space. The cytoplasm contains granular endoplasmic reticulum (ER), rootlets (RL), mitochondria (M), and lysosomes (Ly). A fibrillar aggregate showing a lattice-like structure (*large arrow*) is present within the nucleus (Nuc) at the upper left-hand corner of the illustration.

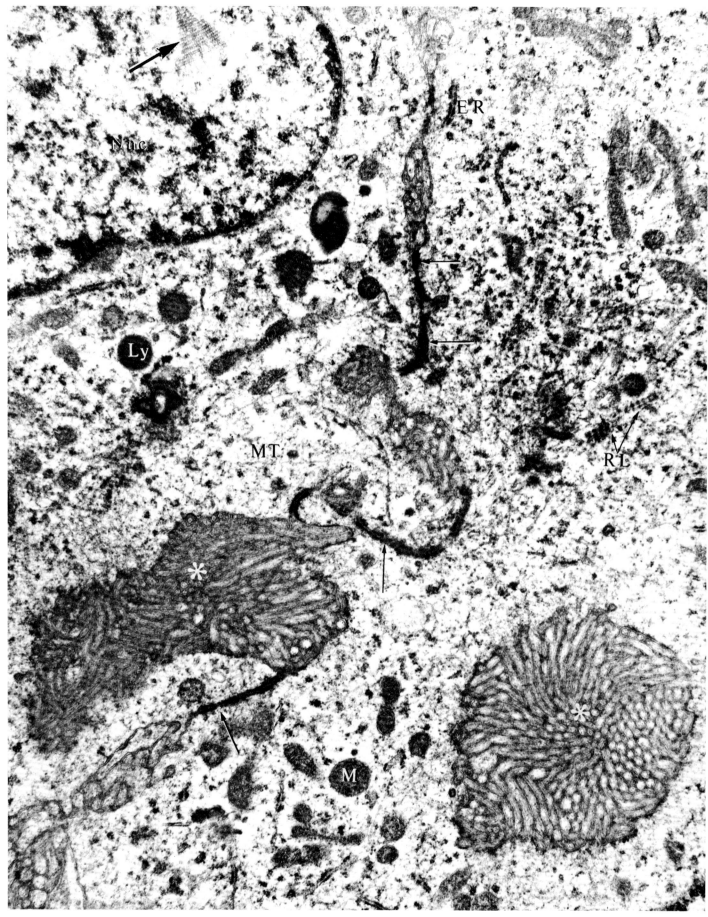

Plate 26   Mag. x24,000

EPENDYMOMA AND OLIGODENDROGLIOMA (CONTINUED)

Plate 27. This micrograph is of the same tumor illustrated in Plate 26. A junctional complex (*arrow*) and an aggregate of microvilli (Mv) are visible. There is a large extracellular space (ES) filled with electron-dense edema fluid. Within the nucleus (Nuc), a lattice-like fibrillar aggregate is present which is shown in the insert at a higher magnification.

The nature and significance of the intranuclear fibrillar aggregates are unknown. Within the present mixed tumor, they were observed in both ependymomatous and oligodendrogliomatous areas. Other investigators have reported similar intranuclear fibrils in oligodendrogliomas, malignant gliomas of other types, reactive astrocytes, and neurons.

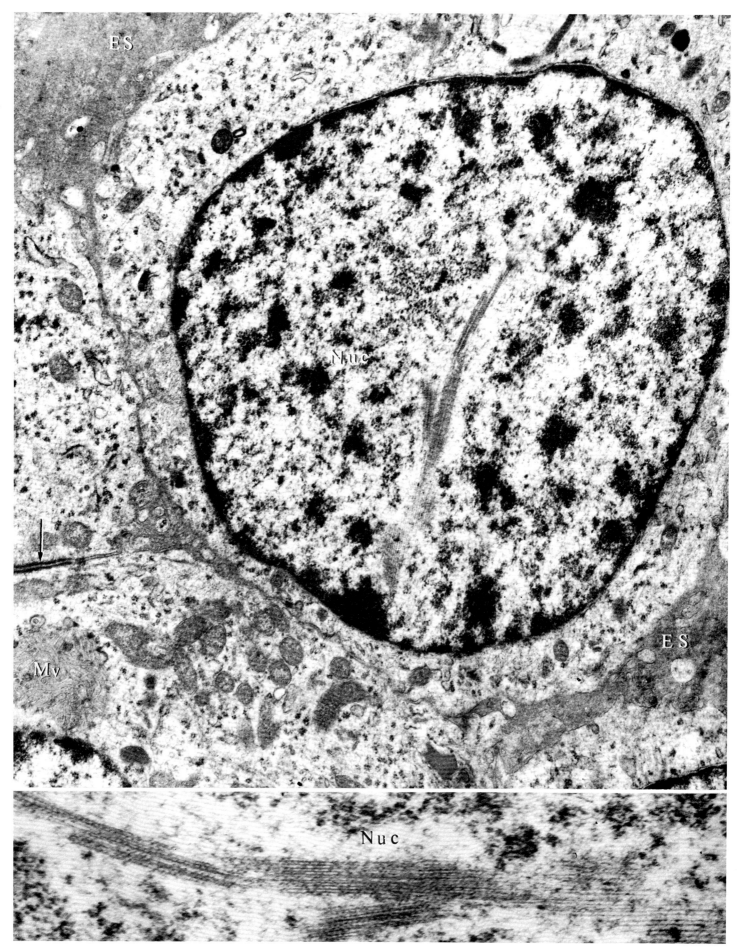

Plate 27   Mag. x30,000.   Insert, mag. x85,000

55

MEDULLOBLASTOMA

Fig. 14. The tumor cells of this medulloblastoma are uniform in size and shape. They have round nuclei and scant cytoplasm. Neither mitoses nor pseudorosettes, common features of this neoplasm, are present in this micrograph. There is an inconspicuous stroma that is limited essentially to perivascular locations. Hematoxylin-eosin stain; mag. x440.

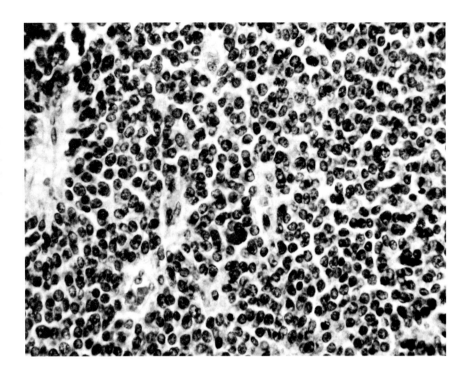

Plate 28. A number of cells and cell processes of this medulloblastoma are crowded together with only narrow extracellular spaces. Collagen fibers are not present. Most tumor cells have round nuclei surrounded by narrow rims of cytoplasm. Microtubules (MT) are scattered in the cytoplasm, but fibrils are not seen. Synapses are absent. Cytoplasmic density is variable, and occasionally elongated nuclei are found in denser cells.

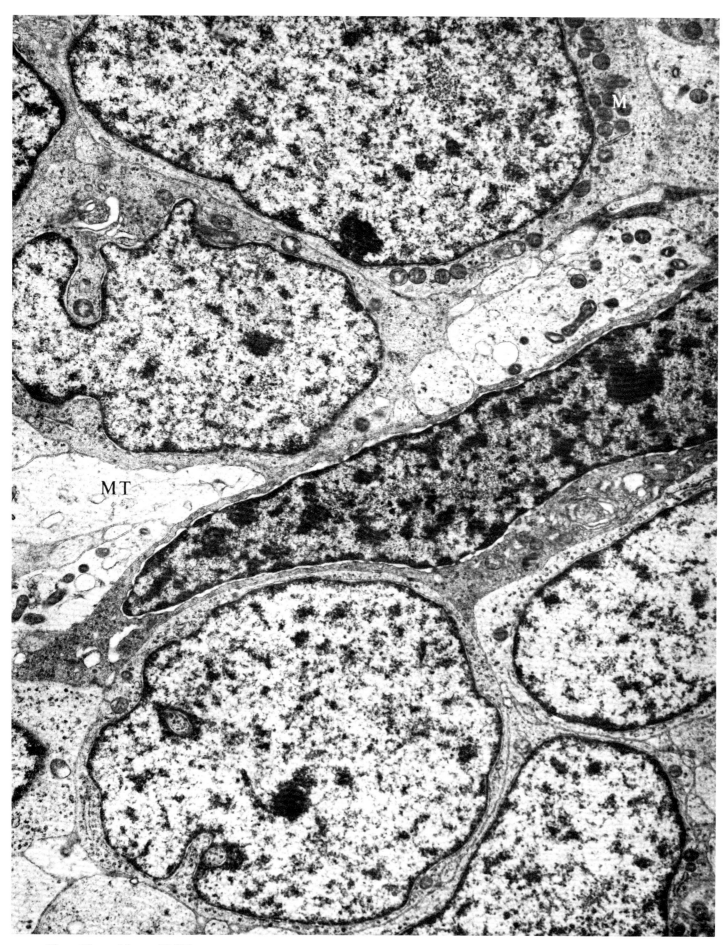

Plate 28   Mag. x12,000

Plate 29. This electron micrograph is from another area of the tumor illustrated in Plate 28. In this field the fine structure is rather similar from cell to cell. Large nucleoli (ncl) are present in two nuclei. Again, the extracellular spaces are very narrow and collagen is absent.

The absence of large extracellular spaces and collagen fibers in this tumor contrasts strikingly with their abundance in cerebellar sarcoma (cf. Plates 31, 32, and 33).

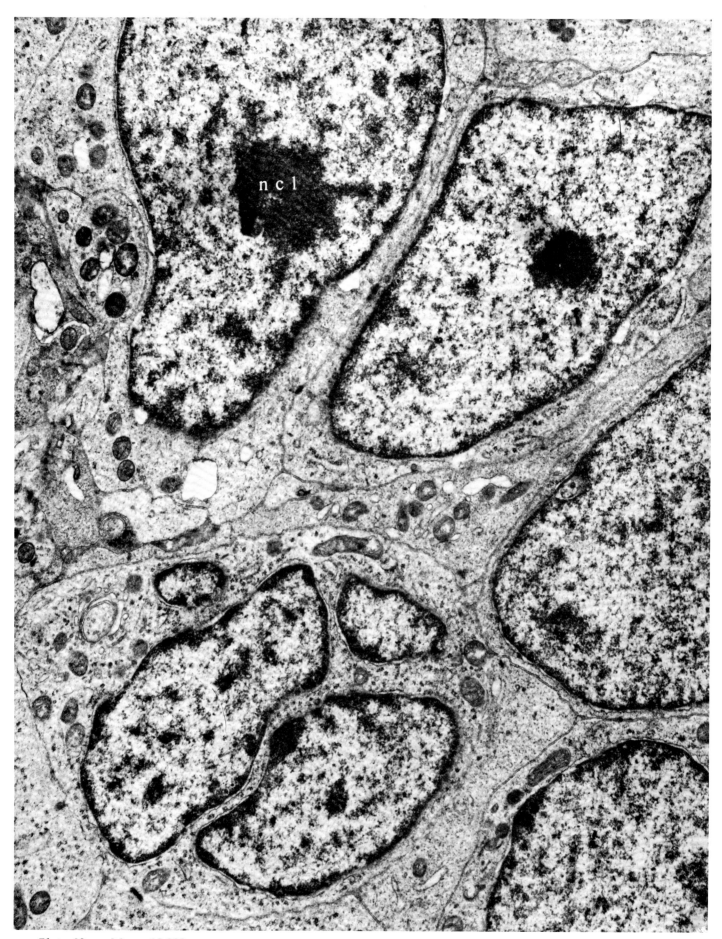

ncl

Plate 29   Mag. x12,000

Plate 30. Electron micrograph of a tumor cell in a medulloblastoma undergoing mitotic division. Dense chromosomes and the oriented microtubules (MT) of the spindle apparatus are visible. No nuclear membrane remains to separate the chromosomes from the cytoplasm organelles such as mitochondria (M). Mitotic figures are frequently encountered in this tumor even in the relatively small samples examined in the electron microscope.

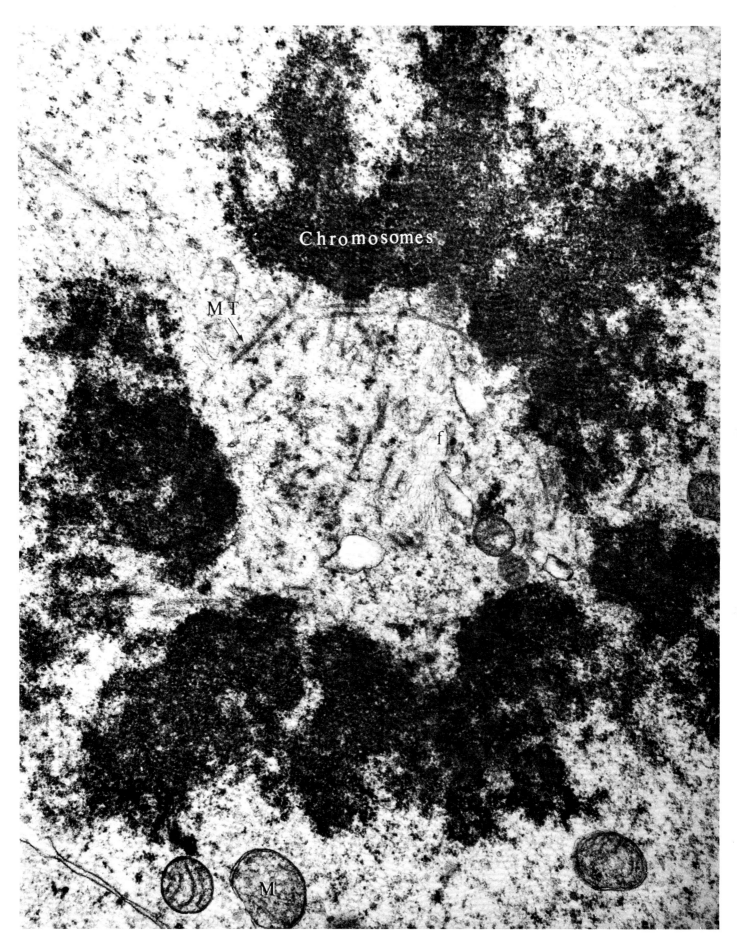

Plate 30   Mag. x35,000

Fig. 15. Columnar and papillary arrangements of tumor cells in a cerebellar sarcoma. Between the columns of cells there is a fine reticulin that is demonstrable to best advantage in silver-impregnated preparations. The reticulin fibers in this tumor are part of the neoplasm even when it is confined to the cerebellar parenchyma, and are not produced only in response to invading neoplastic cells in the leptomeninges. Hematoxylin-eosin stain; mag. x325.

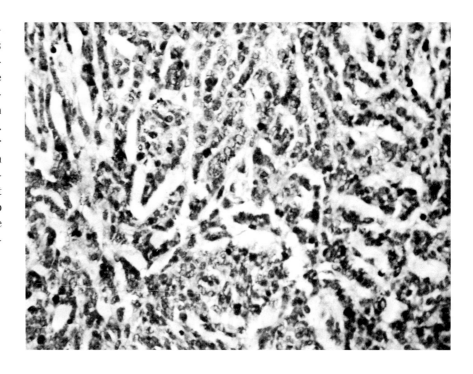

Plate 31. A portion of a chain or column of tumor cells is seen within a large extracellular space (ES) that contains many collagen (Col) bundles. The nuclei are surrounded by narrow rims of dark cytoplasm containing mitochondria and occasional dense bodies (D). Cell processes (Pr) extend into the extracellular space. Intercellular junctional complexes are not present.

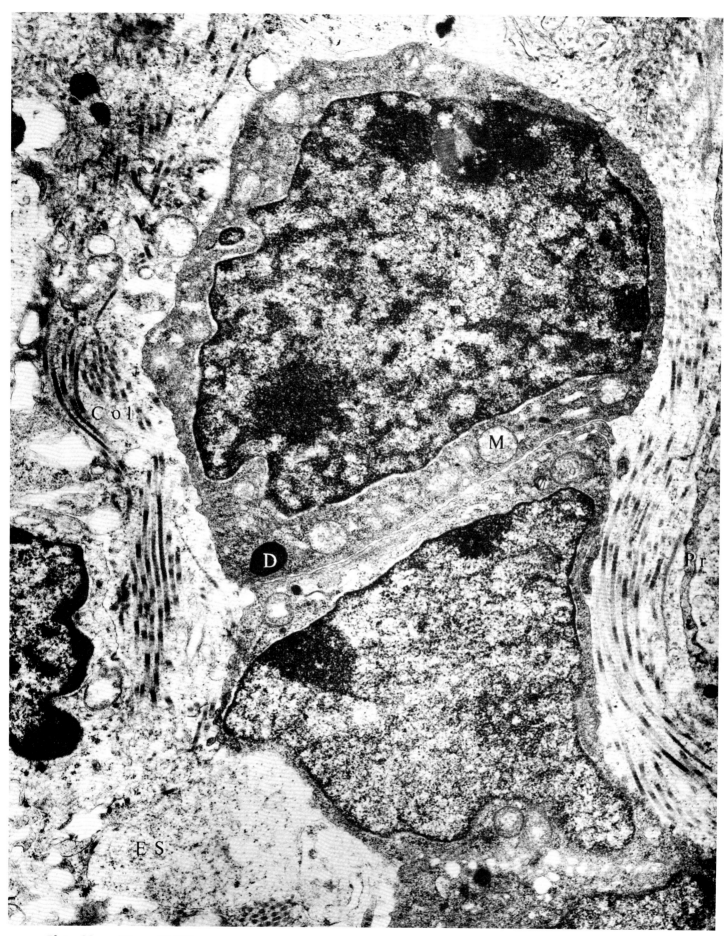

Plate 31   Mag. x25,000

Plate 32. Three widely separated cells in the tumor are present near a blood vessel whose lumen (L), endothelial lining (End), and basement membrane (BM) are seen in the right lower corner of the micrograph. These cells are surrounded by large extracellular spaces (ES) that contain collagen (Col) and a cell process. The cell in the center contains an irregular nucleus and distended rough endoplasmic reticulum (ER) within a dense cytoplasmic matrix. A centriole is also present in this cell.

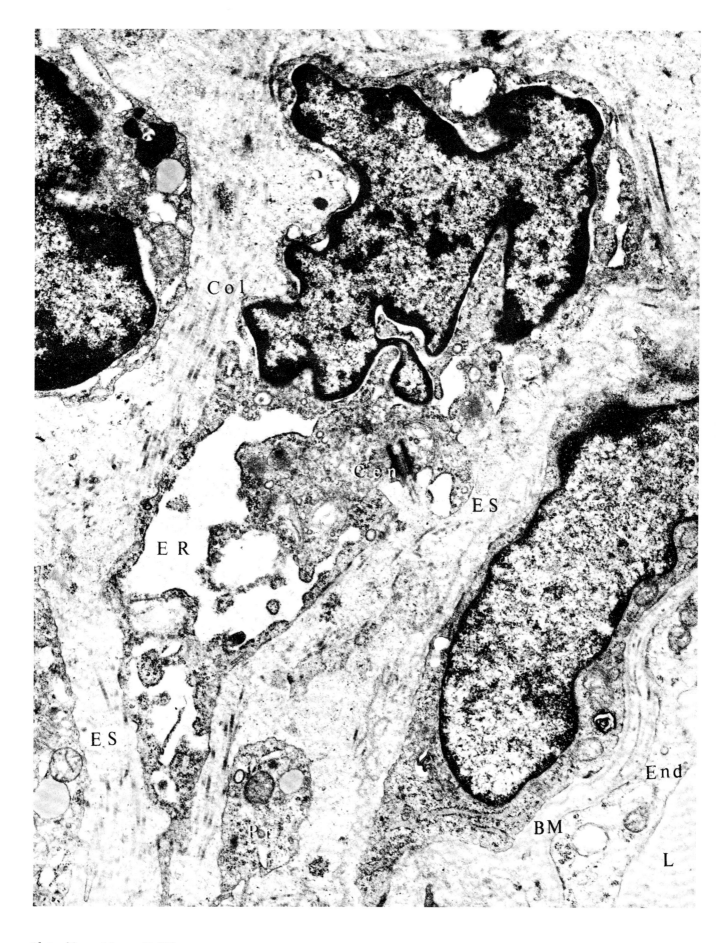

Plate 32 Mag. x21,000

65

Fig. 16. Photomicrograph of a cerebellar sarcoma that contains a dense spherical mass of tumor cells in the center of the illustration. This "glomerular" arrangement of cells is devoid of reticulin, in contrast to the surrounding tumor whose cells form a delicate fibrillar stroma. Hematoxylin-eosin stain; mag. x350.

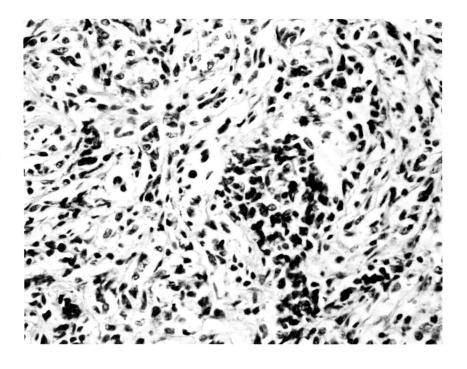

Plate 33. This electron micrograph is of a section through a "glomerular" formation (cf. Fig. 16) in which reticulin was absent. The tumor cells are rather compactly arranged and show a tendency towards chain formation (cells numbered 1, 2, 3, and 4). The extracellular space is narrow but in part appears beaded due to artifactitious alterations that have resulted from necrosis and attendant poor preservation of the plasma membranes. A similar effect of necrosis is the indistinct boundary between the collagen (Col) -containing extracellular space in the lower left-hand corner of the micrograph and the adjacent cell.

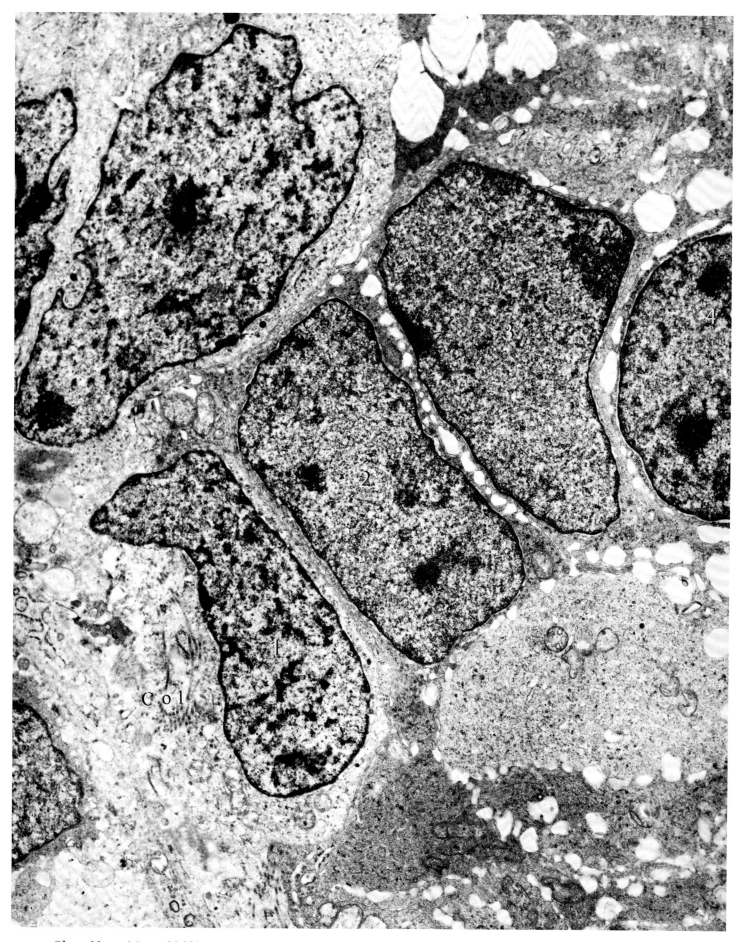

Plate 33   Mag. x16,000

MENINGIOMA

Fig. 17. This photomicrograph is of a classical meningioma with several meningeal whorls and one psammoma body. Hematoxylin-eosin stain; mag. x420.

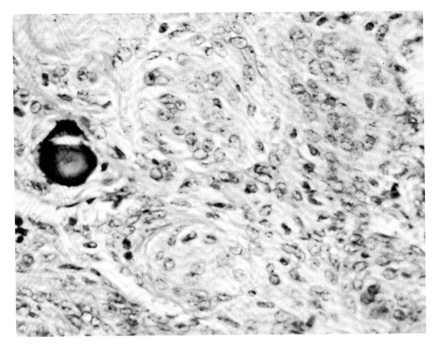

Fig. 18. Meningocytes with intranuclear "inclusions." Several nuclei have clear centers ringed by chromatin material that lies against the inner side of the nuclear membranes. Hematoxylin-eosin stain; mag. x720.

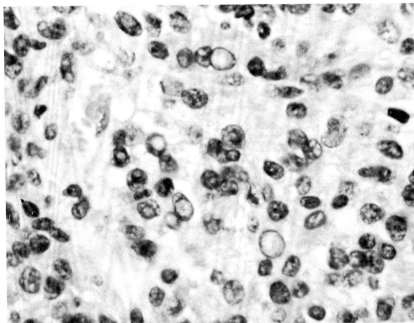

Plate 34. The tumor cells and their attenuated processes are compactly arranged, but small extracellular spaces (ES) are occasionally seen. The nuclei, some with prominent nucleoli (ncl), are often indented so that, as in the upper portion of the micrograph, a cytoplasmic invagination may appear to be intranuclear. This intranuclear "inclusion" is surrounded by both complete cell and nuclear membranes and contains mitochondria (M) and a Golgi apparatus (G). Dense glycogen granules (Gly) are present in the cytoplasm of several tumor cells. The cell surfaces are irregular.

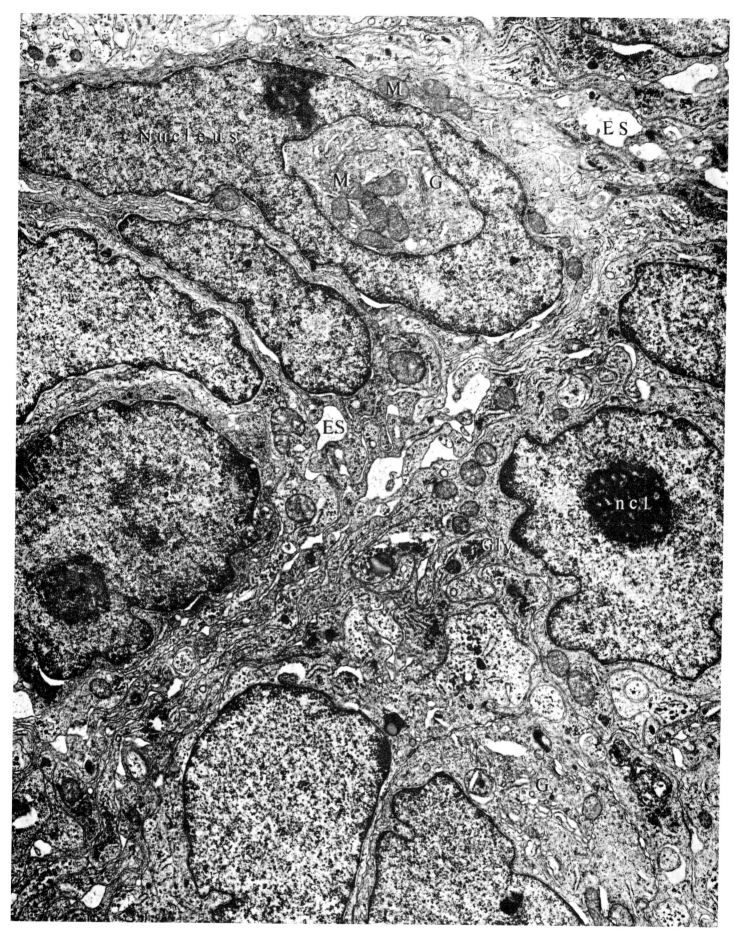

Plate 34   Mag. x19,000

69

Fig. 19. Photomicrograph of meningocytes under high magnification. The cell in the center has an intranuclear cytoplasmic inclusion. Hematoxylin-eosin stain; mag. x1800.

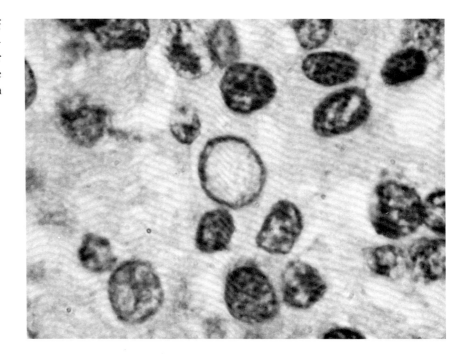

Plate 35. A higher magnification of the same tumor illustrated in Plate 34. The large, irregularly shaped nucleus in the center of the micrograph has two cytoplasmic inclusions. Several closely apposed cell processes (1, 2, 3, 4, and 5), often containing fine fibrils (f) and microtubules (MT), lie adjacent to the cell body.

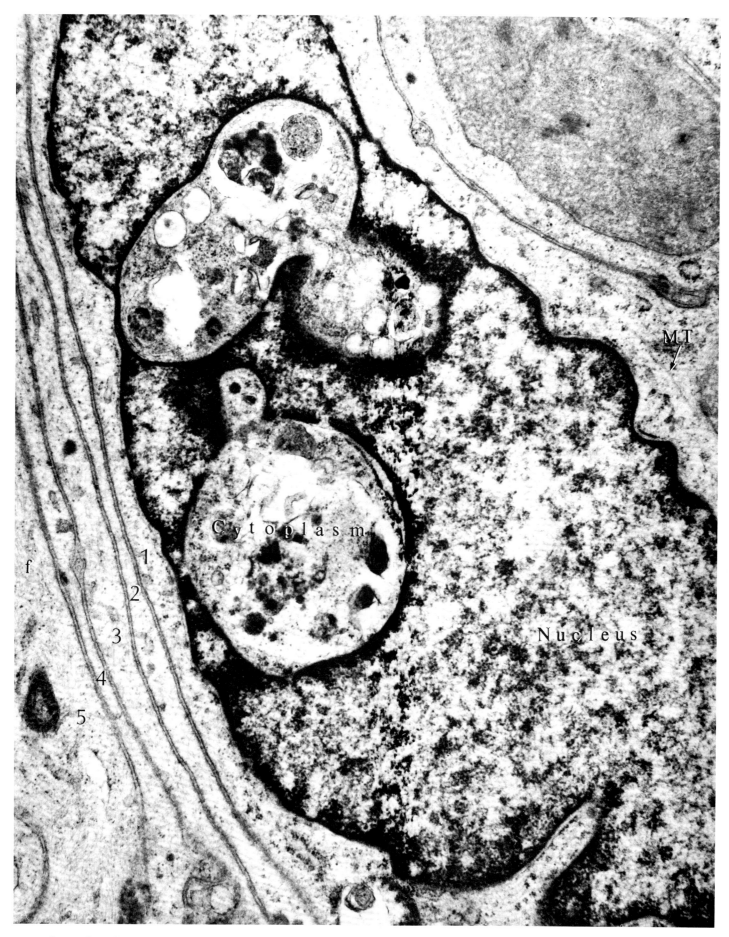

Plate 35   Mag. x42,000

Plate 36. This micrograph illustrates the abundant attenuated cell processes which are often joined by junctional complexes (*arrowheads*), one of the characteristic features of meningiomas. The extracellular spaces are narrow and, in contrast to nerve sheath tumors of the peripheral nervous system, basement membranes are usually not present. Prominent centrioles (Cen), Golgi apparatuses (G), and mitochondria (M) are crowded in the cytoplasm. Obvious, well-developed nucleoli (ncl) are present in two of the nuclei (Nuc).

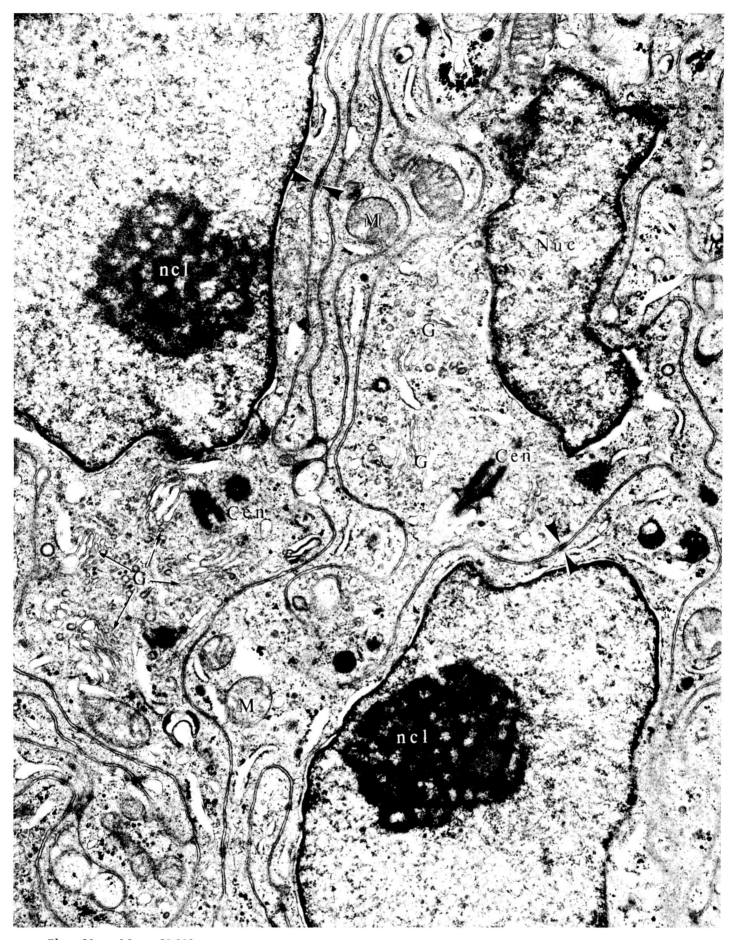

Plate 36   Mag. x30,000

Fig. 20. Photomicrograph of a psammoma body in a meningioma. Note the prominent lamination. Hematoxylin-eosin stain; mag. x720.

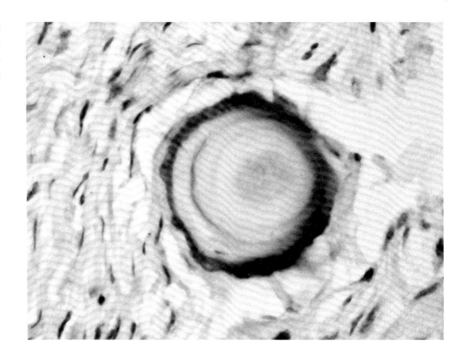

Plate 37. A psammoma body contains a central core of electron-dense spicules, presumably calciferous, surrounded by alternating concentric layers of extracellular spaces filled with collagen fibers and cell processes. Blood vessels, often the origin of psammoma bodies, are not visible in this field. Apparently, then, these bodies have other sites of origin.

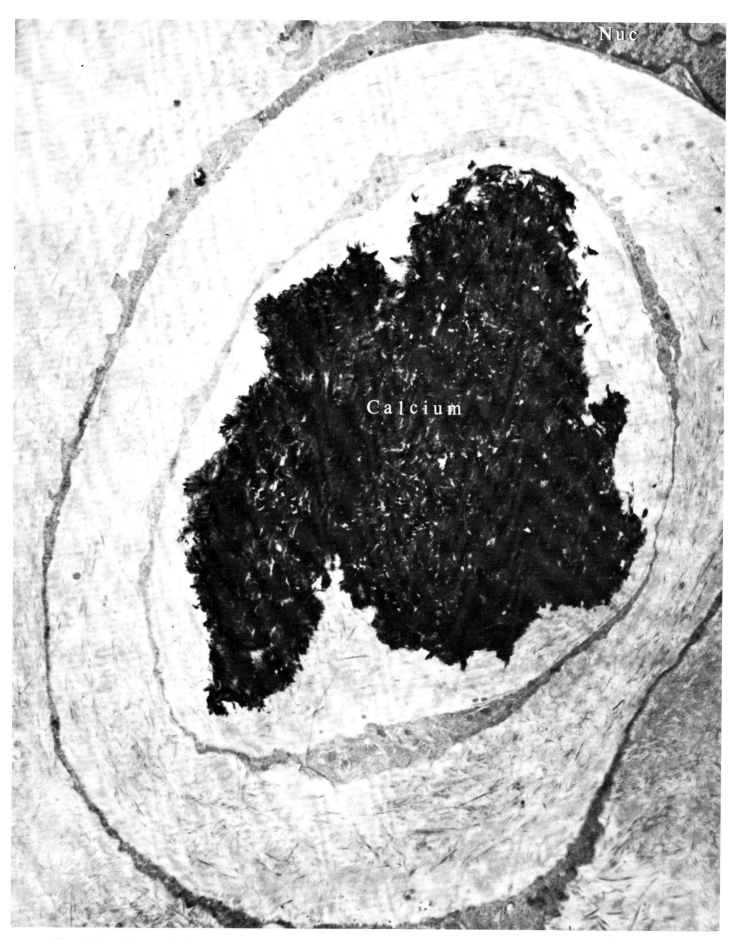

Nuc

Calcium

Plate 37   Mag. x9000

Plate 38. A portion of a psammoma body similar to that illustrated in the previous electron micrograph (Plate 37). Surrounding the dense calcium core, concentric layers of large, collagen-containing extracellular spaces (ES) alternate with sheets of cell processes (Pr). At the periphery of the body (lower right corner) there are seen numerous closely apposed cell processes (1 to 19).

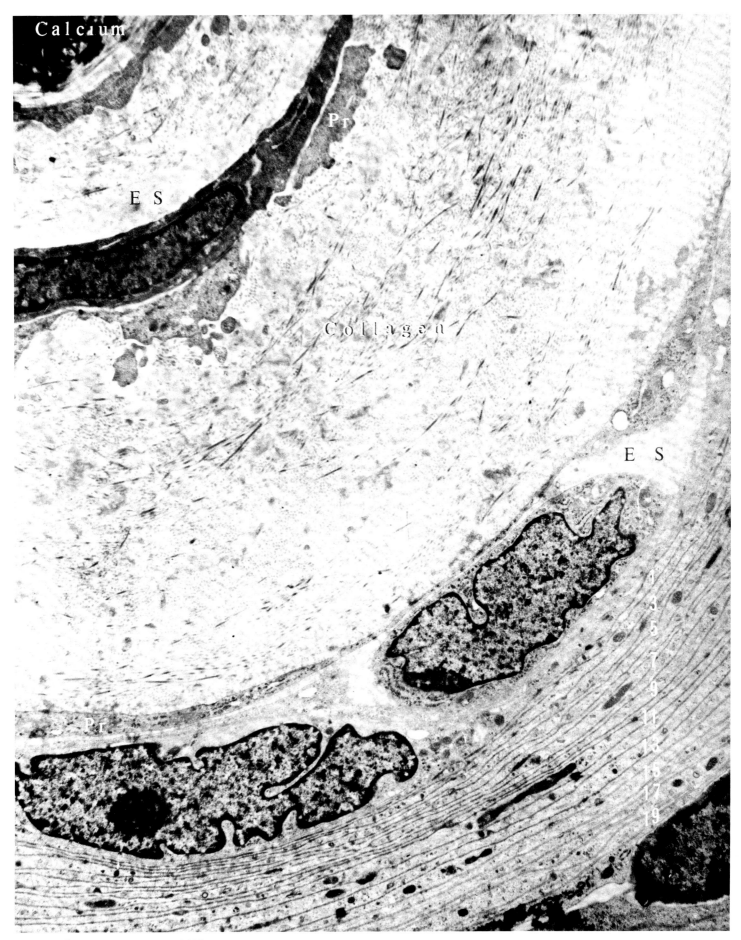

Plate 38   Mag. x14,000

Plate 39.   In some meningiomas the extracellular spaces (ES) contain unusually wide collagen fibers (Col). In this micrograph the fibers measure approximately 1000 Å in diameter, as opposed to the 400 Å of most collagen samples. An adjacent tumor cell contains abundant fibrils (f) and glycogen (Gly) granules.

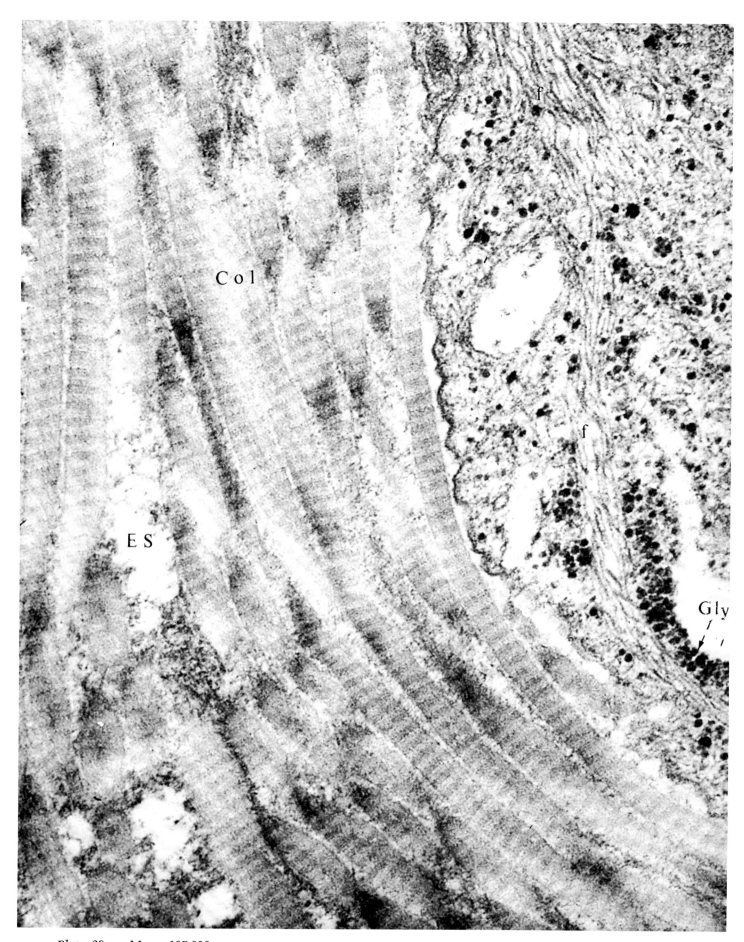

Plate 39   Mag. x105,000

PITUITARY ADENOMAS

Fig. 21. Cuboidal cells are arranged in a glandular pattern in this chromophobe adenoma. Cytoplasmic granules are either absent or so small as to be invisible at this magnification. Hematoxylin-eosin stain; mag. x400.

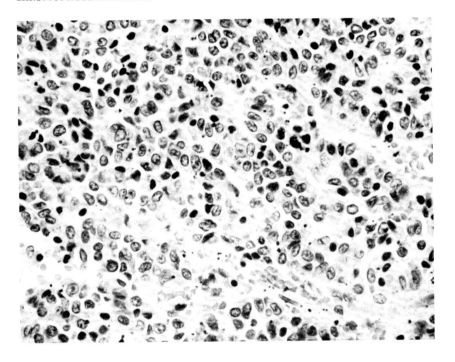

Plate 40. The spherical nucleus of this essentially cuboidal tumor cell is surrounded by a highly vacuolated cytoplasm containing numerous small mitochondria (M). Minute dense secretory granules (SG) and a few scattered larger membrane-bounded lipid bodies (Li) are also present. The sides of this tumor cell abut on other tumor cells with only a narrow extracellular space intervening. The basal portion of the cell rests on a narrow basement membrane which faces a large, dense, collagen-containing extracellular space (ES).

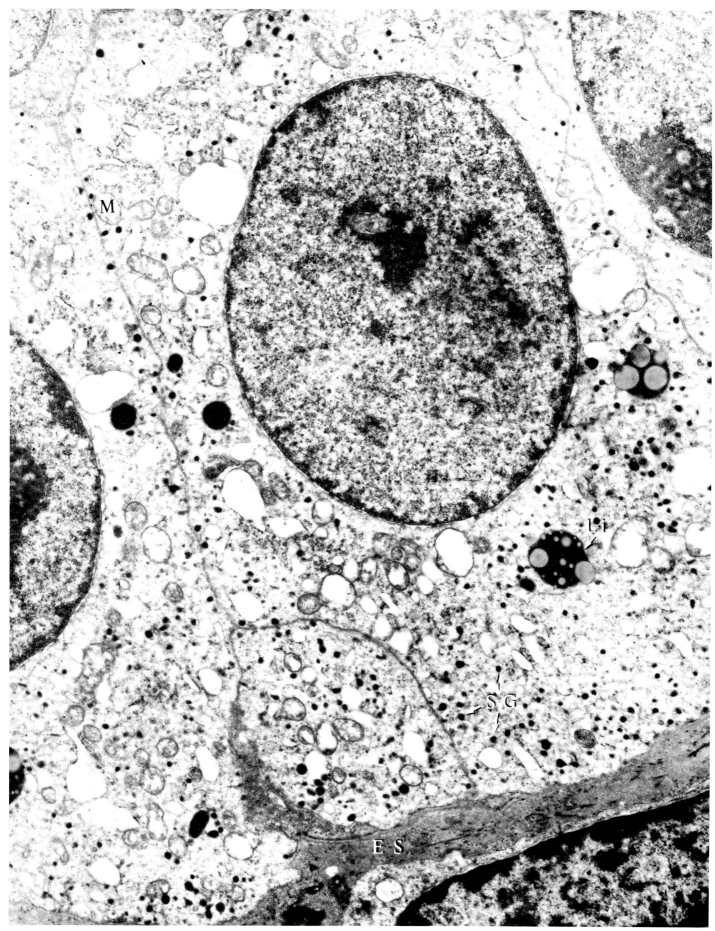

Plate 40   Mag. x12,000

CHROMOPHOBE ADENOMA (CONTINUED)

Plate 41. Higher magnification of a tumor cell similar to that illustrated in Plate 40. Small dense granules (SG) as well as larger lipid bodies are visible. Numerous mitochondria (M) are present of which some apparently contain lipid inclusions (*large arrows*). Small secretory granules (*double arrows*) are scattered throughout the cytoplasm.

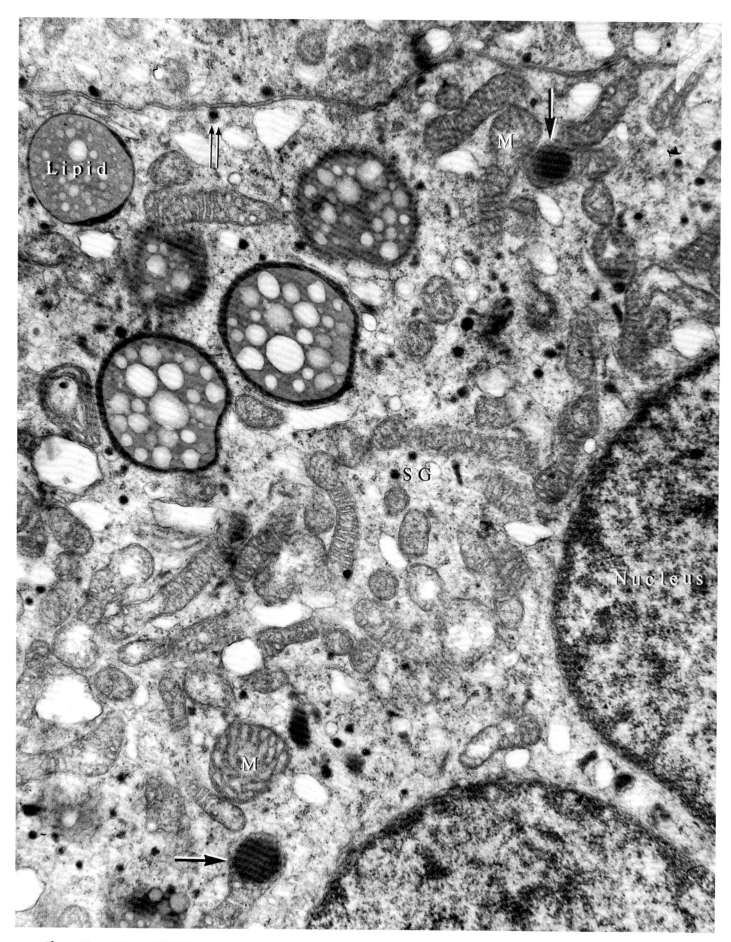

Plate 41   Mag. x37,000

83

EOSINOPHILIC ADENOMA

Fig. 22. The large epithelioid cells are loosely arranged and have prominent cytoplasmic bodies that are deeply eosinophilic (gray in this black and white illustration). Hematoxylin-eosin stain; mag. x400.

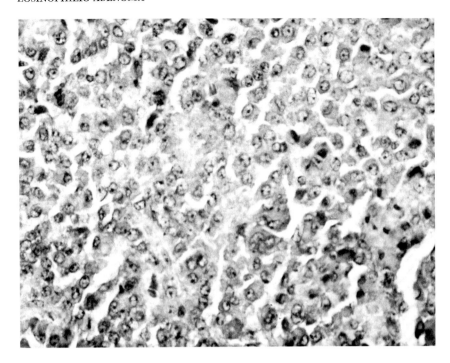

Plate 42. This electron micrograph is of a tumor cell in an eosinophilic pituitary adenoma and illustrates the large number of dense secretory granules that correspond to the eosinophilic granules seen with the light microscope. In addition to occasional mitochondria (M), a well-developed rough endoplasmic reticulum (ER) is present.

The large number and size of the secretory granules in this tumor, as well as the presence of a well-developed endoplasmic reticulum, are in striking contrast to the situation found in chromophobe adenomas.

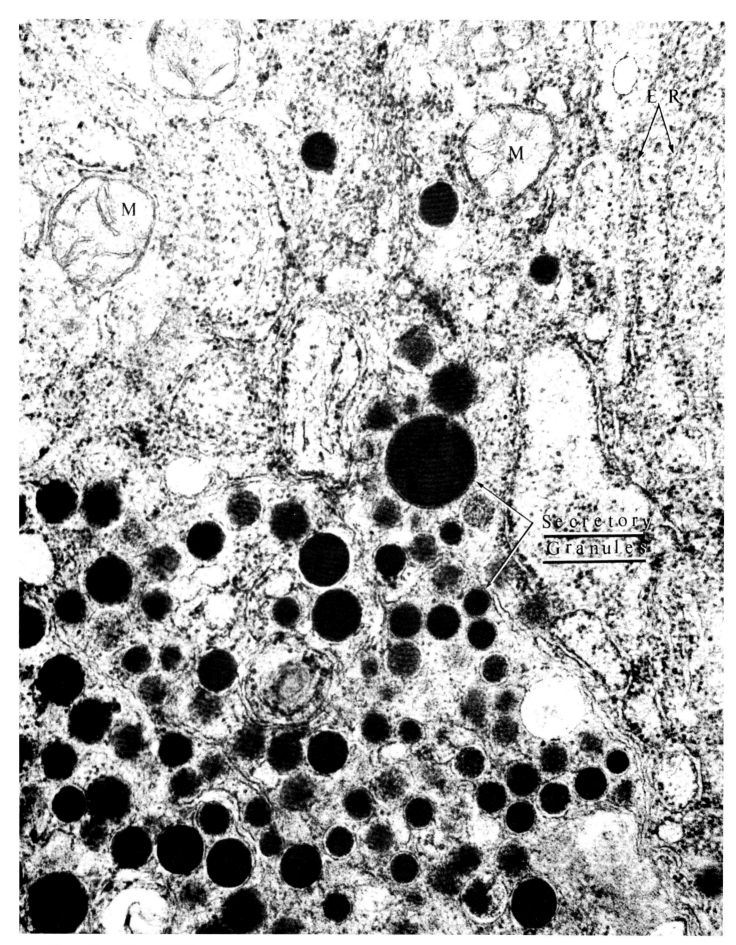

Plate 42   Mag. x55,000

85

CRANIOPHARYNGIOMA

Fig. 23. Multicystic craniopharyngioma with each individual microcyst lined by a single layer of columnar cells. Hematoxylin-eosin stain; mag. x275.

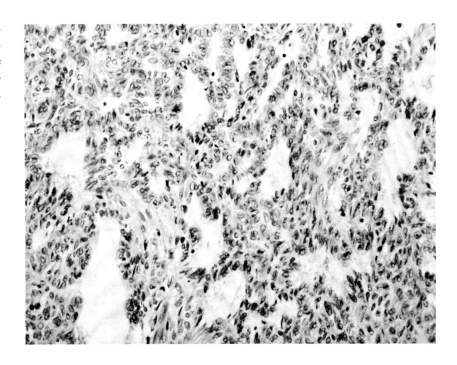

Plate 43. Low-magnification micrograph of a craniopharyngioma whose tumor cells are compactly arranged in the upper portion of the illustration but less so in the lower third. Here there are pockets of extracellular space (ES). The cells are similar throughout the field and all have desmosomes (Des). The area of the tumor illustrated in this micrograph is remarkable for its similarity to the stratum spinosum of the skin.

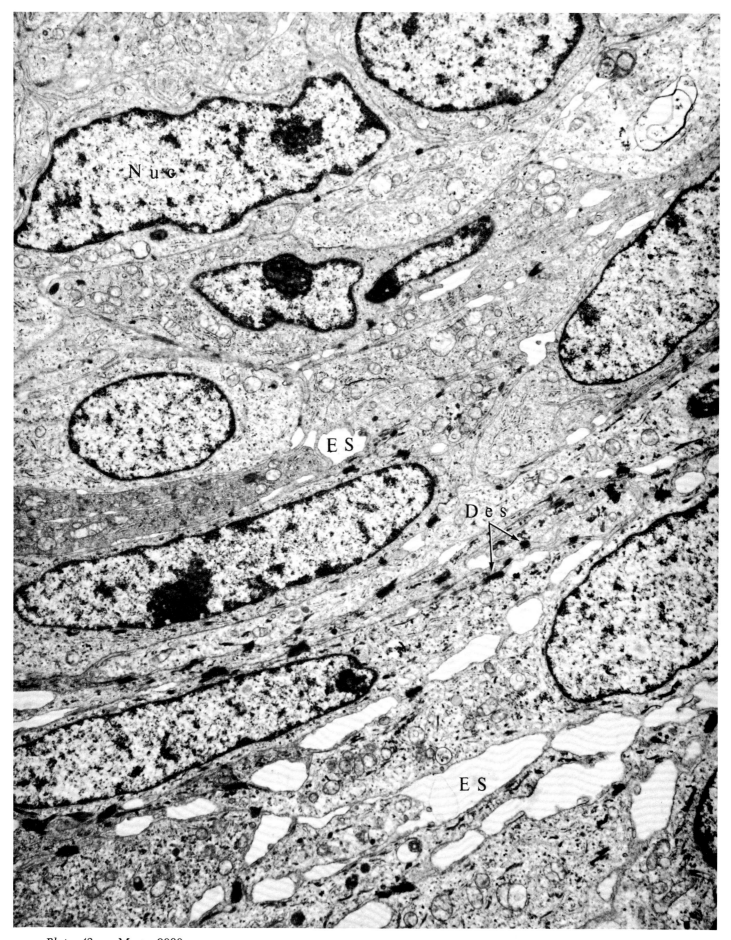

Plate 43   Mag. x9000

87

Fig. 24. Craniopharyngioma of the squamous epithelial type. Note the delicate intercellular bridges between some of the cells. Hematoxylin-eosin stain; mag. x460.

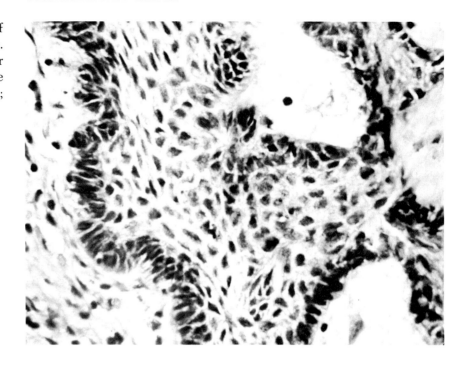

Plate 44. Electron micrograph of a craniopharyngioma showing the conspicuous, well-developed desmosomes (Des) between adjacent cells. The desmosomes consist, in part, of fibrillar material extending for some distance into the cytoplasm. Just beyond their termination, bundles of similar fibrils, the tonofilaments, may be seen (*arrow*). Between the desmosomes, the extracellular spaces (ES) are distended to form small cysts lined by a moderately electron-dense reticulated material. Further distension of the extracellular cysts results in the formation of the multiloculated cavities characteristic of certain craniopharyngiomas.

This electron micrograph is indistinguishable from that of the stratum spinosum of normal skin. The desmosomal junctions correspond to the intercellular bridges seen with the light microscope.

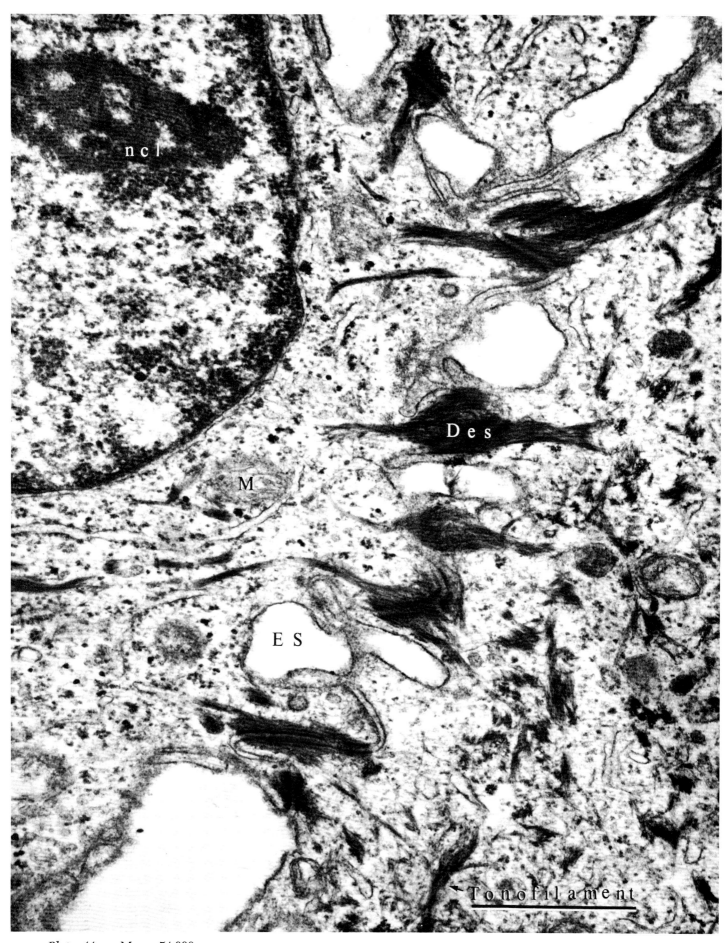

Plate 44   Mag. x54,000

Plate 45. Electron micrograph under high magnification of a Rosenthal fiber within a reactive astrocyte adjacent to a craniopharyngioma. Numerous glial fibrils (f) are in close contact with the dense granular mass that constitutes the Rosenthal fiber.

These fibers have been observed with the light microscope in a variety of conditions including neoplasms as well as inflammatory and degenerative disorders.

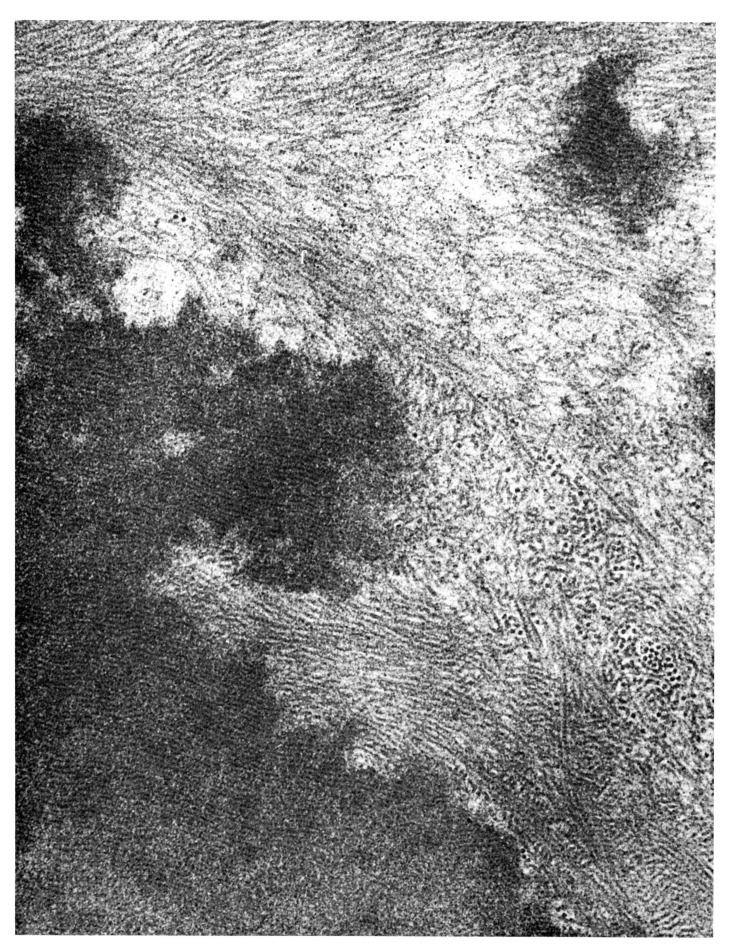

Plate 45   Mag. x120,000

CEREBELLAR
HEMANGIOBLASTOMA

Fig. 25. The tumor is composed of large cells with clear cytoplasm and numerous vascular channels with thin walls. Nests of tumor cells lie between the capillaries. Hematoxylin-eosin stain; mag. x450.

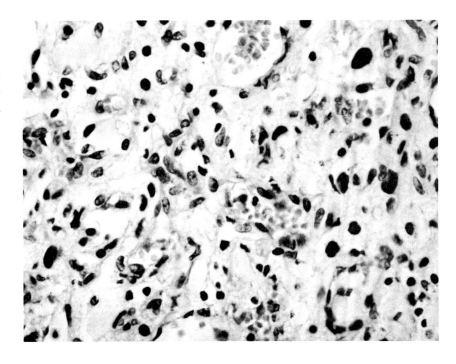

Plate 46. The tumor cell in this micrograph has an irregular nucleus (Nuc) and distended endoplasmic reticulum that forms clear spaces of irregular size and shape in the cytoplasm. Several spheroid, membrane-bounded, dense lipid inclusions can be seen. Frequently the lipid inclusions occupy a large part of the cell volume, rendering the cell highly sudanophilic in frozen sections viewed with a light microscope. The usual paraffin-embedded preparations extract the lipid so that the cells appear clear and empty. The distended endoplasmic reticulum also contributes to the empty appearance of the cell.

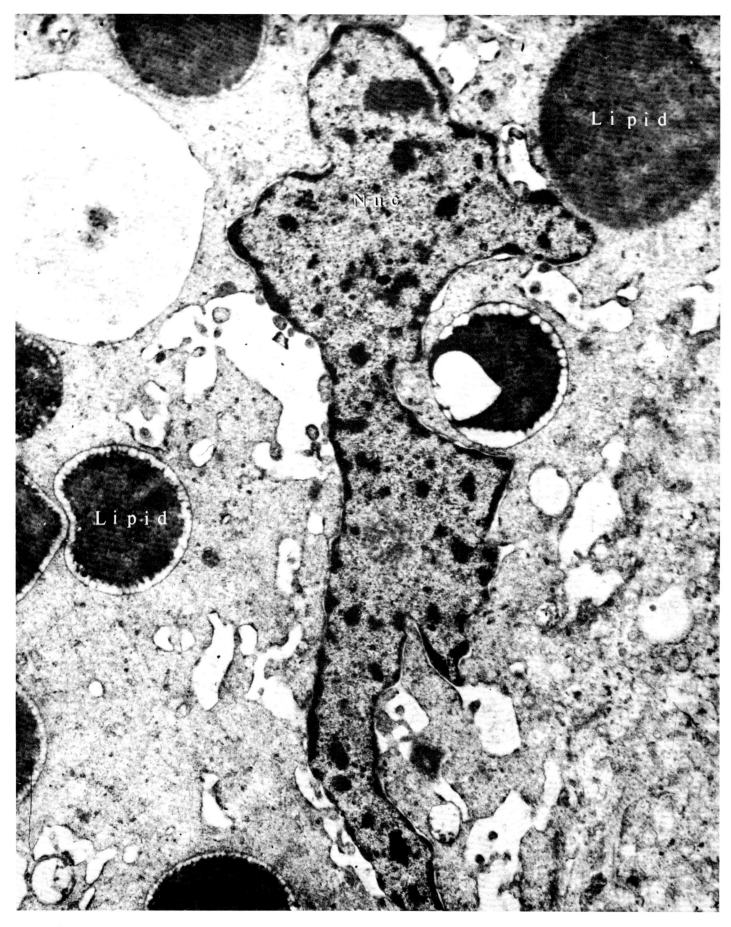

Plate 46   Mag. x31,000

MALIGNANT LYMPHOMA
OF BRAIN

Fig. 26. Photomicrograph of primary malignant lymphoma (lymphosarcoma) involving blood vessel wall, Virchow-Robin space, and adjacent cerebral parenchyma. The tumor cells are mainly of the small round cell (lymphocytic) variety, but larger mononuclear tumor cells (reticulum cells?) are also present. Hematoxylin-eosin stain; mag. x325.

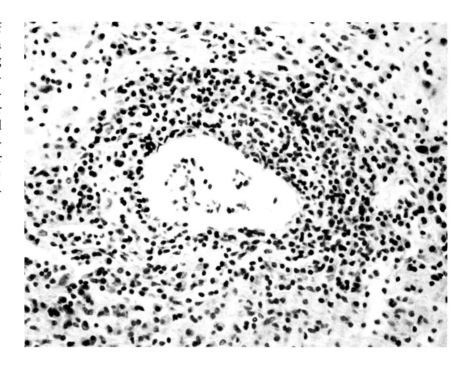

Plate 47. This micrograph is of an essentially spherical tumor cell within a large extracellular space containing a large amount of electron-dense, plasma-like material and many cell processes (Pr). The dense cytoplasm contains an irregular nucleus with prominent chromatin (Chr), scattered mitochondria (M), a centriole (Cen), lysosomes (Ly), a Golgi apparatus (G), endoplasmic reticulum (ER), and numerous free and membrane-associated ribosomes. A nearby cell shows microtubules (MT) in the cytoplasm. The cell surface is decorated with finger-like projections.

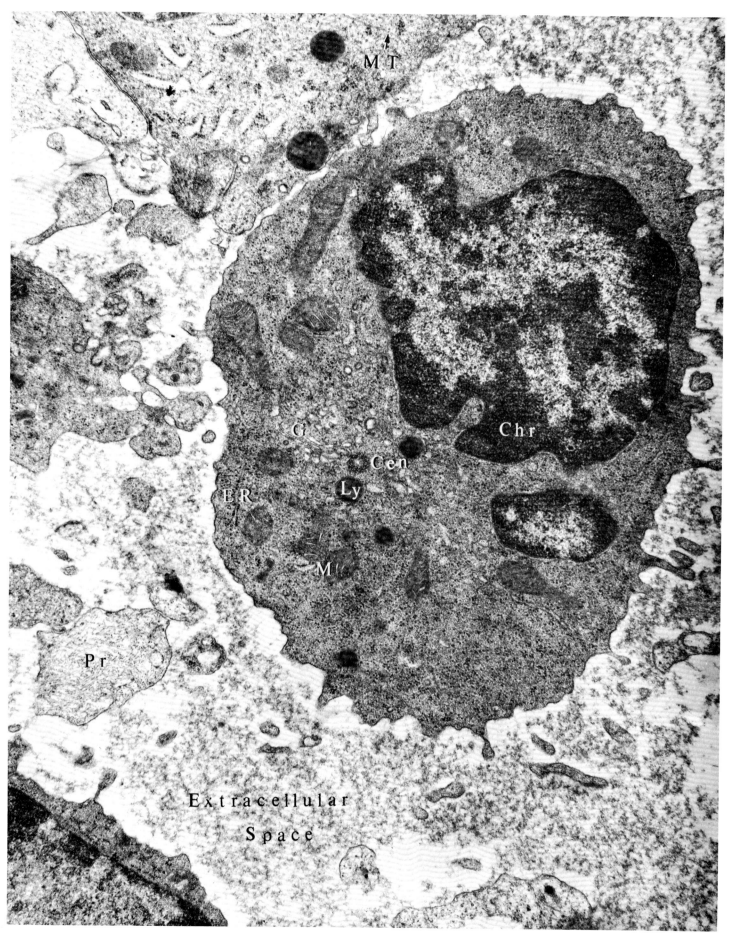

Plate 47   Mag. x30,000

Fig. 27. Tumor cells form a cuff around a cerebral blood vessel and invade the vessel wall as well as the parenchyma. Large neurons can be seen amidst tumor cells on the left side of the figure. Hematoxylin-eosin stain; mag. x400.

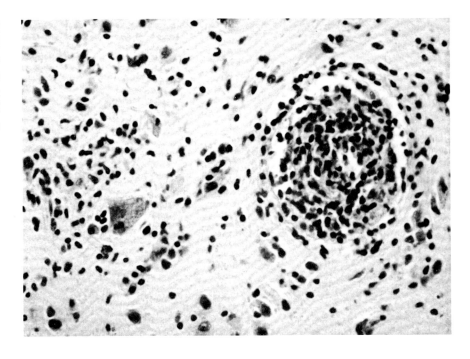

Plate 48. Micrograph of a plasma cell within the same tumor illustrated in Plate 47. This cell is characterized by its well-developed rough endoplasmic reticulum (ER). Margination of the chromatin (Chr) is evident within the nucleus. The cell lies within a large extracellular space (ES) that also contains other cell processes (Pr.)

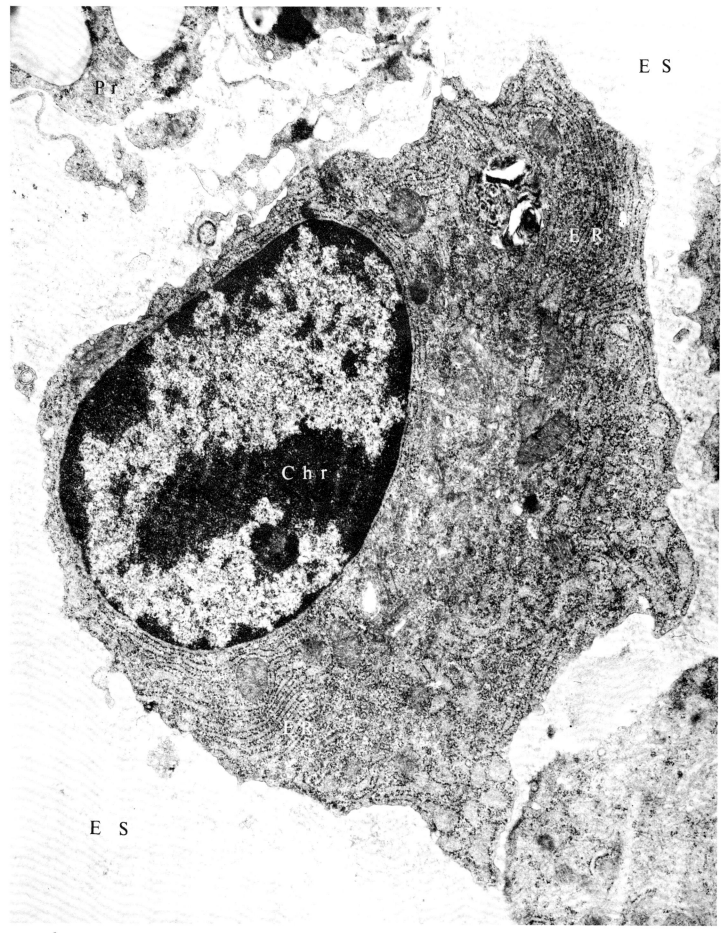

ES

Pr

ER

Chr

ER

ES

Plate 48   Mag. x25,000

NEURILEMOMA

Fig. 28. Photomicrograph of an acoustic neurilemoma showing the parallel arrangement of elongated tumor cells that also form incomplete palisades. Hematoxylin-eosin stain; mag. x150.

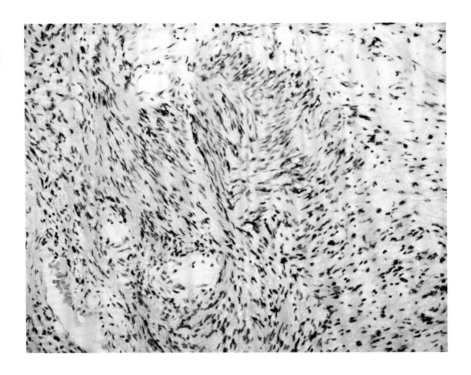

Plate 49. Under low magnification this electron micrograph of the acoustic neurilemoma illustrated in Fig. 28 shows the parallel arrangement of spindle-shaped cells and their processes (Pr). The latter are generally coated by bands of basement membrane (BM). Wide extracellular spaces (ES) are present.

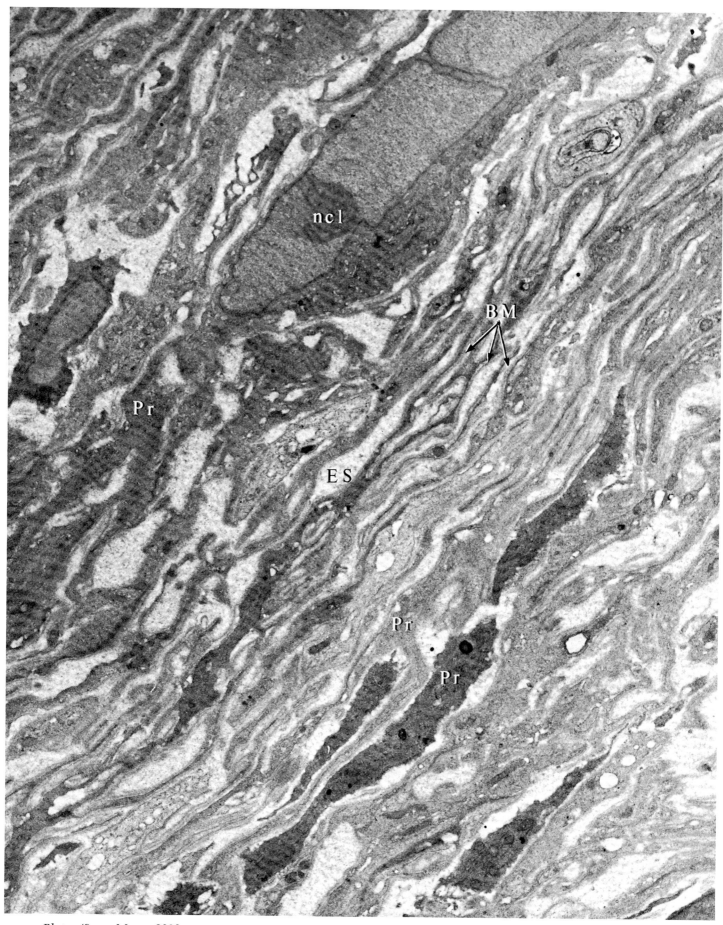

Plate 49   Mag. x8000

Plate 50.   Higher magnification of an area of the neurilemoma illustrated in Plate 49. Most of the cellular processes (Pr) are coated with base-ment membrane (BM) and are separated by collagen-containing extra-cellular spaces (ES).

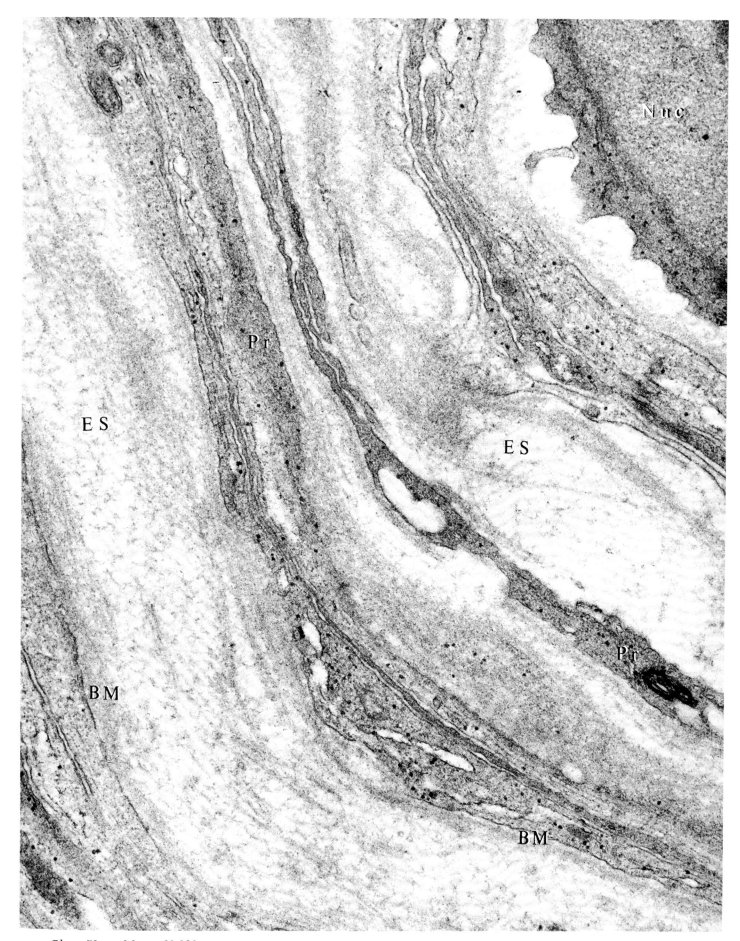

Plate 50   Mag. x60,000

101

Plate 51. Cross section of a tumor cell with an irregular nucleus (Nuc) whose membrane shows evidence of infolding. The structure in the center of the nucleus is a cytoplasmic extension. The cytoplasm is narrow and dense but contains mitochondria (M). Basement membrane (BM) coats the surface of the cell. Bundles of collagen fibers (Col) in cross section are present in the extracellular spaces (ES).

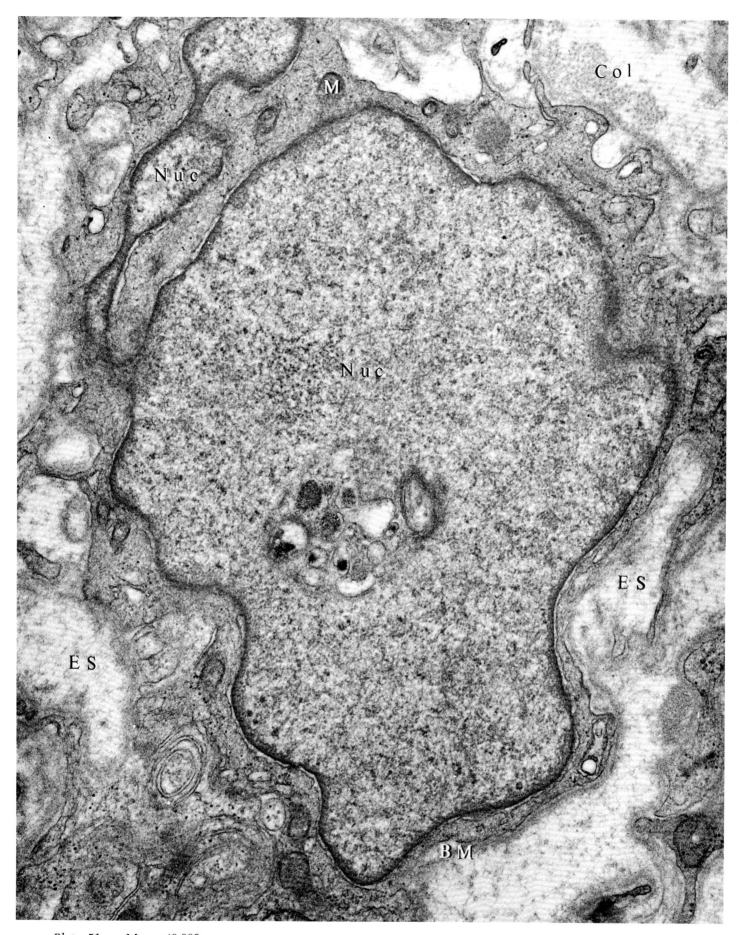

Plate 51   Mag. x40,000

Fig. 29. Palisading of tumor
cells in an acoustic neurilemona.
The elongated cells lie within
and are separated by a fibrillary
stroma. Hematoxylin-eosin stain;
mag. x250.

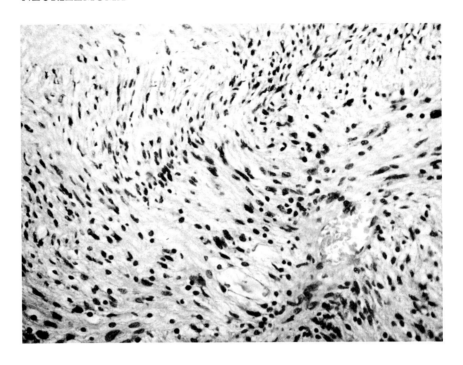

Plate 52. This micrograph is of a tumor cell from the neurilemoma
shown in Fig. 29. The cell is coated with basement membrane (BM)
and is surrounded by a wide extracellular space containing numerous
collagen fibers. Dense bodies (D) are present in the cytoplasm.

Note: The origin of the tumor cells of a neurilemoma is controversial.
Some regard the cells as of fibroblastic origin because of the presence of
collagen fibers. Others, because fibroblasts are not normally coated
with basement membrane, consider the tumor to be derived from Schwann
cells. These cells, moreover, may also be capable of producing collagen.
Finally, the cells lining the inner and outer surfaces of the normal perineurium are coated with basement membrane.

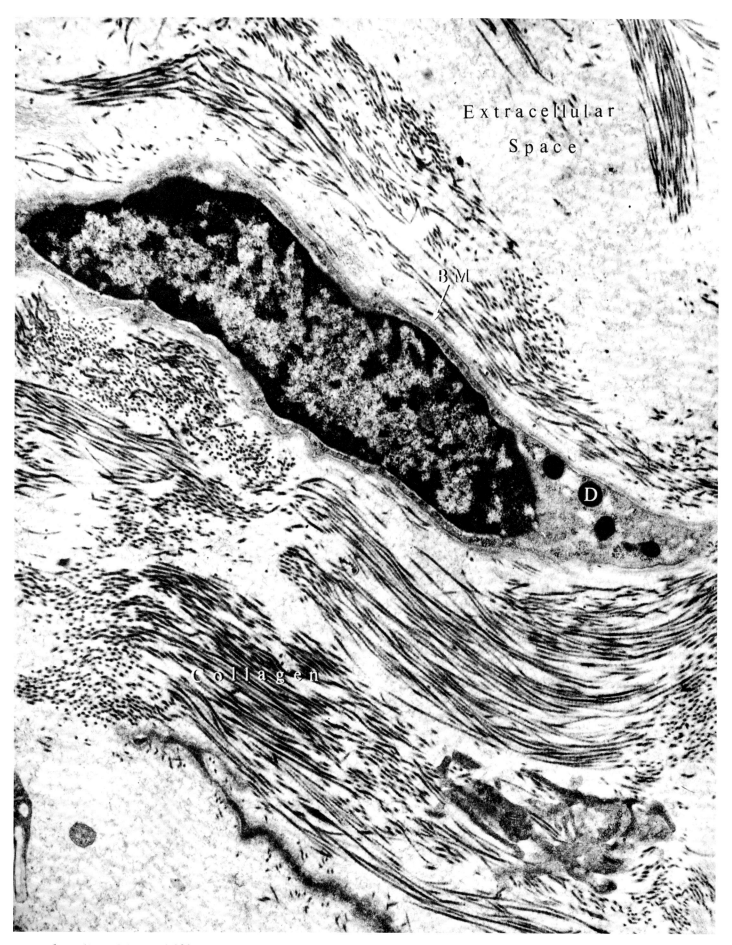

Extracellular

Space

BM

D

Collagen

Plate 52   Mag. x12,000

105

Fig. 30. "Foam" cells in an a-
coustic neurilemoma. These are
fat-laden, sudanophilic cells. Hematoxylin-eosin stain; mag. x250.

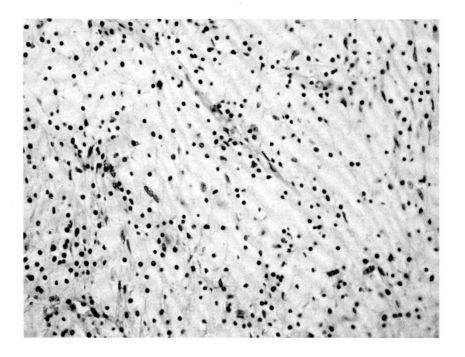

Plate 53. top. The extracellular space in this neurilemoma contains a
spindle-shaped structure that has regular striations with a periodicity of
1000–1200 Å. (Structures of this kind were originally described in acoustic
Schwannomas by Sarah Luse and have since been called "Luse bodies."
Identical structures have been observed in other neoplastic and nonneoplastic pathologic conditions, in Meissner's tactile corpuscles, and in
such nonneuronal sites as Descemet's membrane.)

Bottom. Some of the "foam" cells shown in Fig. 30 contain laminated
structures or "myelin figures," illustrated in this micrograph.

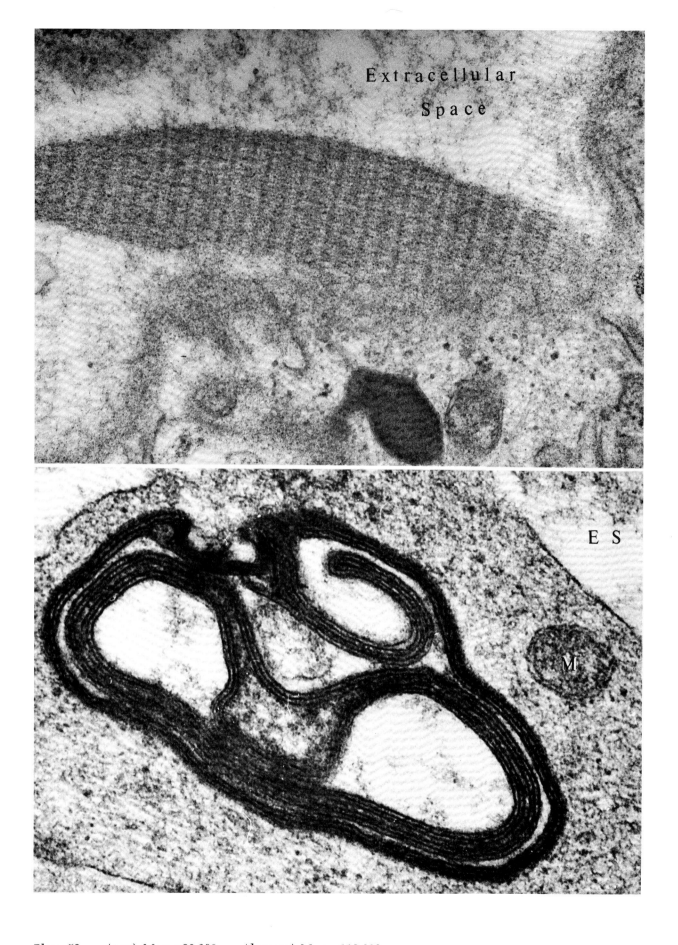

Extracellular
Space

E S

M

Plate 53   (*top*) Mag. x80,000.   (*bottom*) Mag. x118,000

METASTATIC TUMORS

EPIDERMOID PULMONARY CARCINOMA

Fig. 31. Solid nests of epithelial neoplastic cells lie in a desmoplastic stroma within the brain. Hematoxylin-eosin stain; mag. x250.

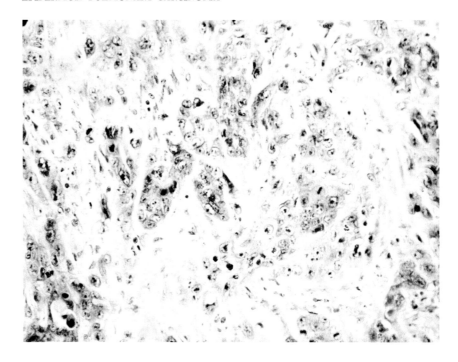

Plate 54. Electron micrograph of a tumor cell shown in Fig. 31. Its nucleus (Nuc) is highly irregular in shape, and its cytoplasm is filled with compactly arranged organelles. The rough endoplasmic reticulum (ER) is particularly well developed, and there are many tonofibrils (TF). An occasional electron-dense lipid droplet is present, as well as a mitochondrion (M).

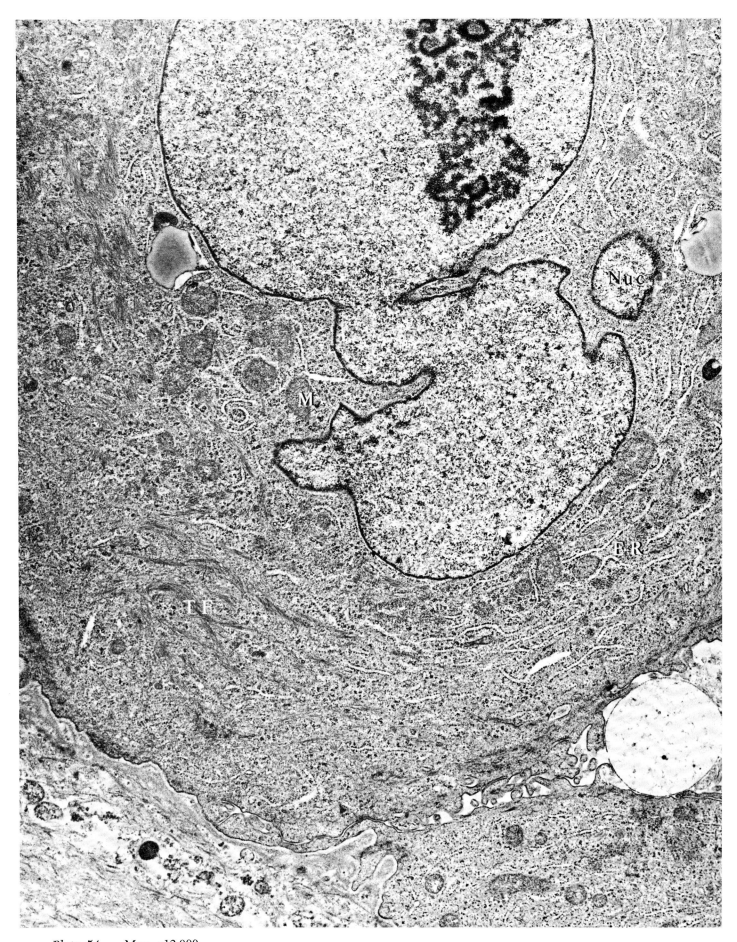

Plate 54   Mag. x12,000

EPIDERMOID PULMONARY CARCINOMA (CONTINUED)

Plate 55. In the same tumor illustrated in Fig. 31 and Plate 54, a small extracellular cyst is shown in the upper left-hand corner of this micrograph. It is lined by cells with short microvilli (Mv). The cells have irregular nuclei, well-developed rough endoplasmic reticulum (ER), and tonofibrils (TF). Intercellular junctions are characterized by numerous desmosomes. Microvilli are also present within the small pockets of extracellular spaces (ES) between desmosomes. A higher magnification of a desmosome is seen in the inset.

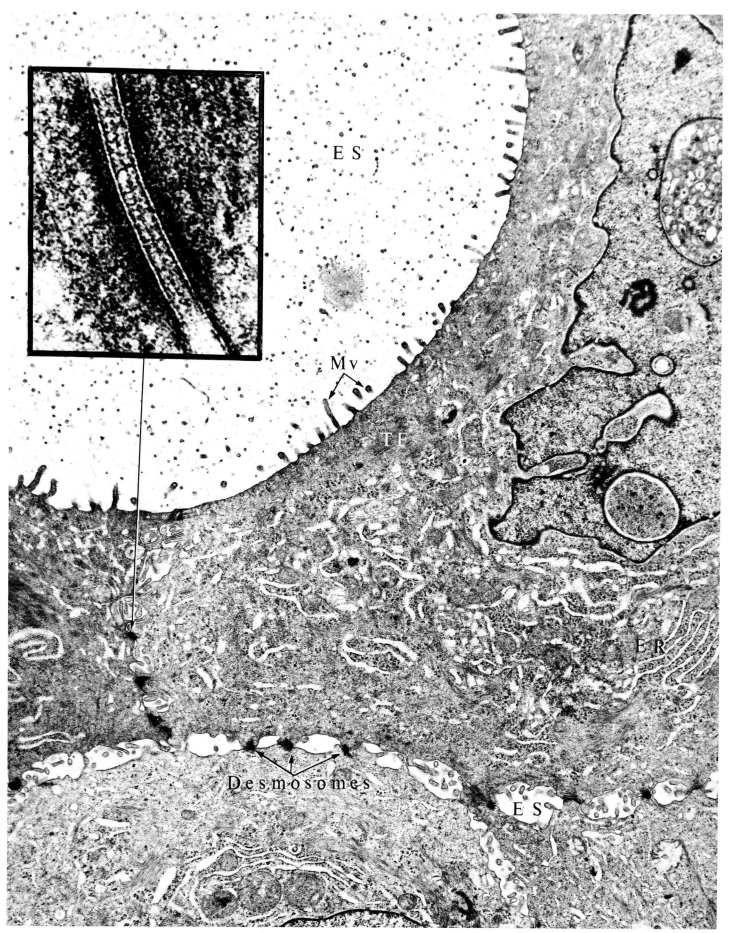

E S

M v

T F

E R

E S

Desmosomes

Plate 55   Mag. x20,000.   Insert, mag. x224,000

111

EPIDERMOID PULMONARY CARCINOMA (CONTINUED)

Plate 56. Higher magnification of the luminal surface of a tumor cell lining a cystic extracellular space (ES) similar to the one illustrated in Plate 55. The microvilli (Mv), seen in both cross and longitudinal planes, are coated with a fine fibrillar material which is attached to the external leaflet of the plasma membrane. Well-developed desmosomes (Des) are present between adjacent cells.

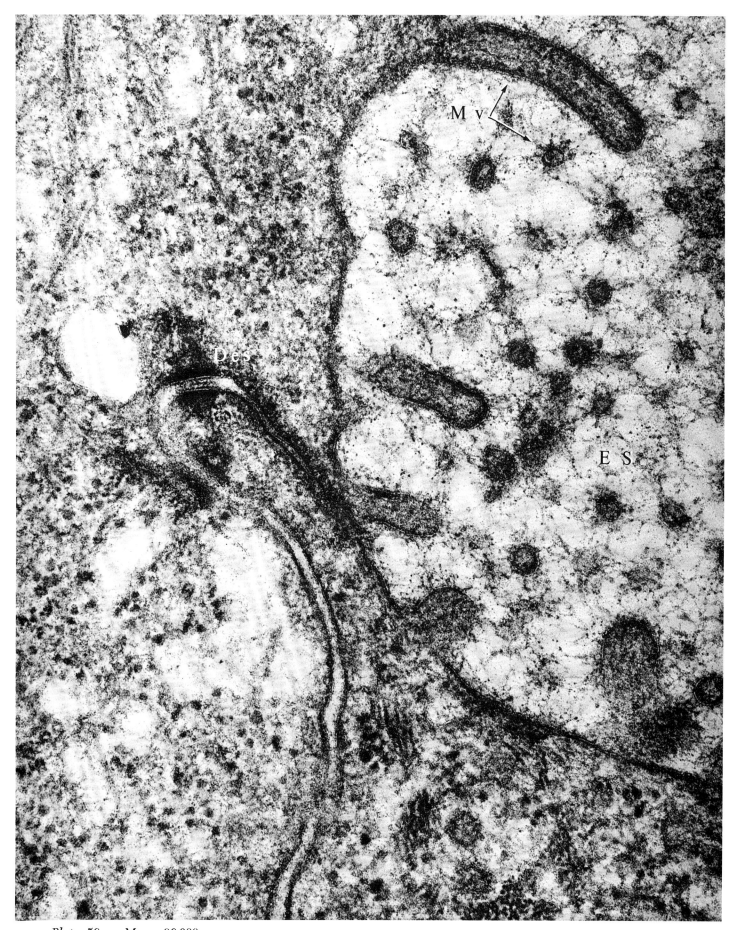

Plate 56   Mag. x96,000

CLEAR CELL CARCINOMA OF KIDNEY

Fig. 32. The nest of clear cells of this renal metastatic carcinoma in the brain has some resemblance to the tumor cells in cerebellar hemangioblastoma (cf. Fig. 25). The cells are plump and have clear cytoplasm and dark round nuclei. Hematoxylin-eosin stain; mag. x450.

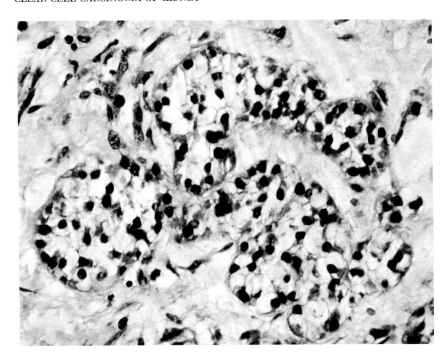

Plate 57. Compactly arranged tumor cells contain large cytoplasmic areas devoid of the usual organelles but containing, instead, numerous scattered electron-dense granules. These areas in the cytoplasm constitute the bulk of the cell volume. The cell periphery, and especially the perinuclear zones, contains denser cytoplasm that holds the usual organelles such as the Golgi apparatus (G). The nuclei are somewhat irregular in shape and contain prominent nucleoli (ncl).

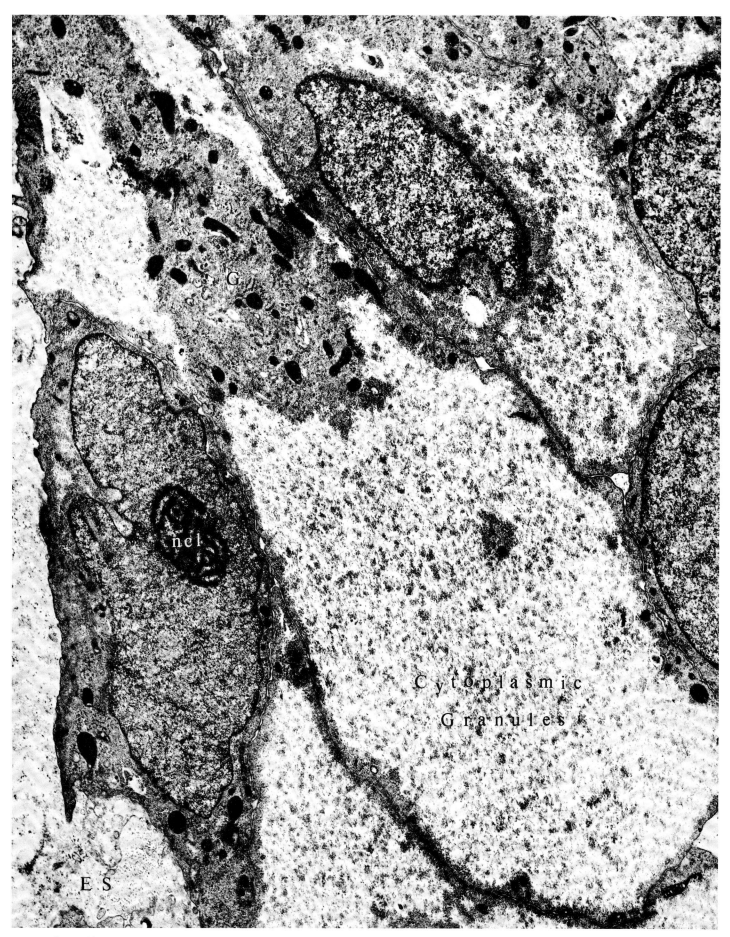

Plate 57   Mag. x20,000

CLEAR CELL CARCINOMA OF KIDNEY (CONTINUED)

Plate 58. top. High magnification of the cytoplasmic granules (CG) shown in Plate 57. These granules measure between 150–250 Å in diameter and are identified as glycogen. A narrow extracellular space is visible near the right edge of the micrograph.

Bottom. View of a peripheral portion of a tumor cell containing fibrils (f) and rough endoplasmic reticulum (ER).

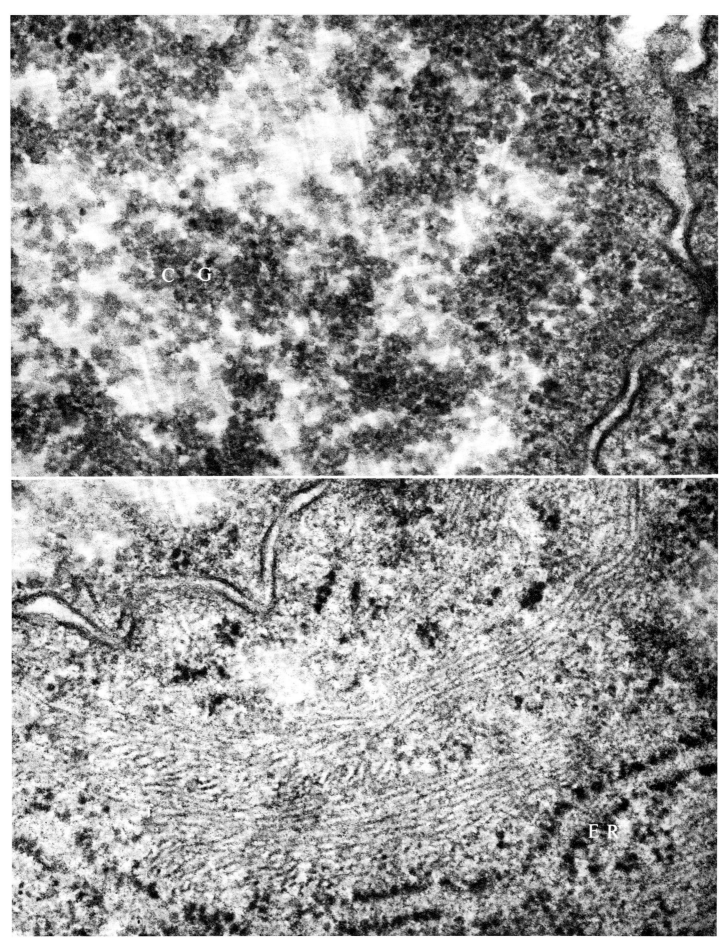

Plate 58   (*top*) Mag. x128,000.   (*bottom*) Mag. x128,000

117

CRYPTOCOCCAL GRANULOMA

Plate 59. Micrograph of a nonneoplastic macrophage harboring three cryptococci near an irregularly shaped nucleus. The cell is necrotic, but certain organelles such as lipid droplets and filaments are still discernible. The capsular material surrounding each cryptococcal organism is well preserved, although the cytoplasm is in a poor state of preservation. The arrangement of the outer capsule and the cell wall of the cryptococci are similar to that seen in the live organism.

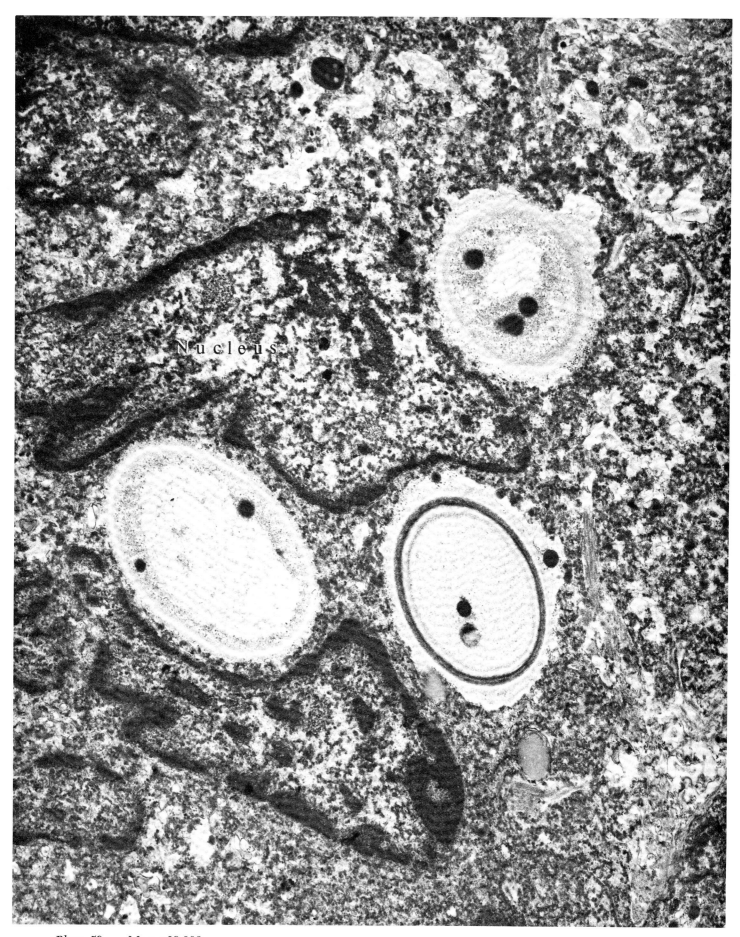

Nucleus

Plate 59   Mag. x28,000

SPINAL EPITHELIAL CYST

Problem: A 44-year-old man showed signs and symptoms indicating compression of the lower portion of the spinal cord and conus medullaris. A large intradural and extramedullary thin-walled cyst, which was attached to the cord substance, was removed at operation.

The cyst wall consisted of a single layer of cuboidal cells, often ciliated (*Fig. 33*). Because of its occurrence within the central nervous system and the presence of cilia, it was suspected that the cyst was of ependymal origin.

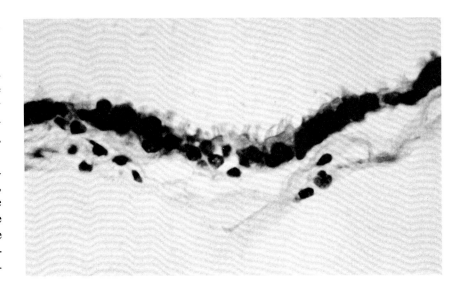

Plate 60. Electron micrograph of the cyst wall shows ciliated as well as nonciliated cells. The basal portions of the cells are covered, unlike most ependymal cells, by a basement membrane (BM) which lines a collagen-containing (Col) extracellular space. The nonciliated cells send projections of microvilli (Mv) into the lumen of the cyst. Although not visible in this micrograph, many nonciliated cells contain variable numbers of secretory granules.

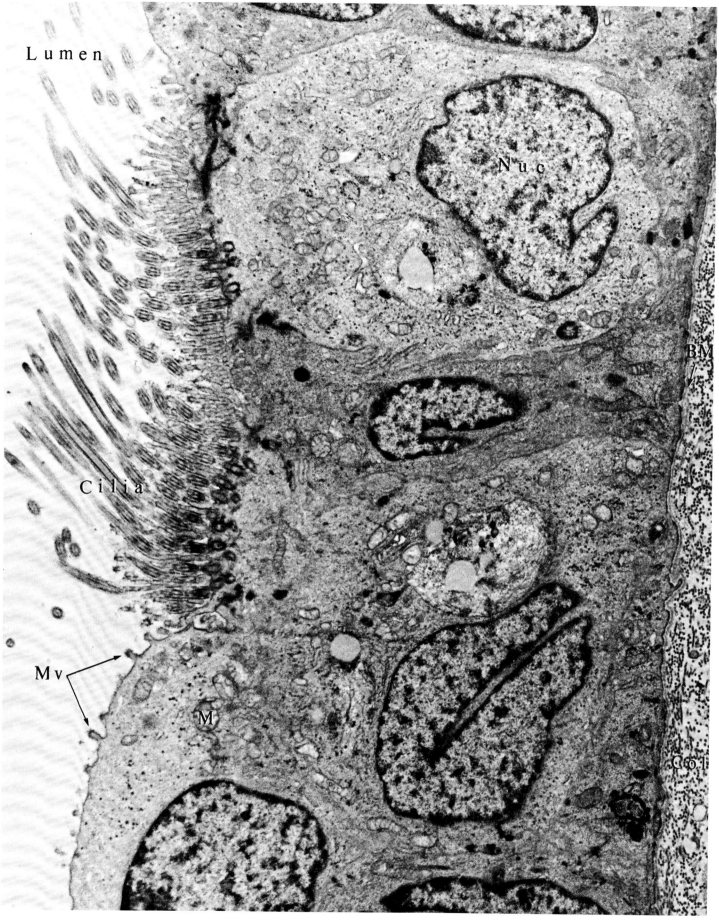

Lumen

Nuc

BM

Cilia

Mv

M

Col

Plate 60   Mag. x10,000

Plate 61. High magnification of the microvilli (Mv) of a nonciliated cell. Unlike cilia or microvilli of ependymal cells, these microvilli are coated with a granulofibrillary material.

Conclusion: On the basis of the material that coats the microvilli of the nonciliated cells lining the cyst, and the secretory granules, there is greater similarity between the epithelium of this cyst and respiratory epithelium than ependyma.

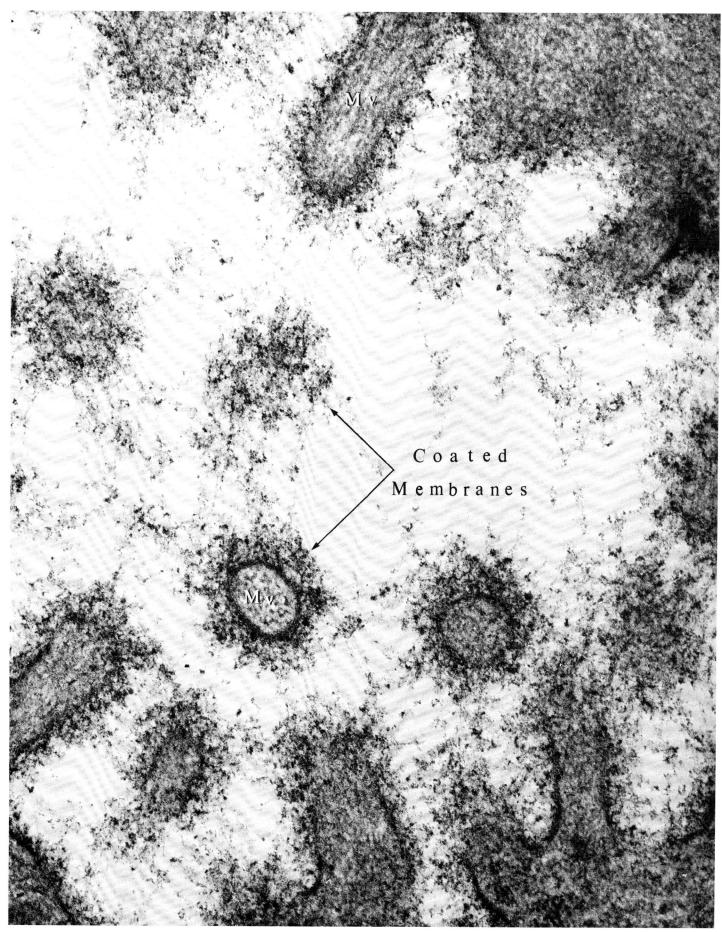

Mv

Coated
Membranes

Mv

Plate 61   Mag. x128,000

REFERENCES

GENERAL

ANDREWS, J. M., and SEKHON, S.S.: Varieties of intranuclear filamentous aggregates in cerebral neurons. Bull. Los Angeles Neurol. Soc. 34:163-174, 1969.

CAUNA, N., and Ross, L.L.: The fine structure of Meissner's touch corpuscles of human fingers. J. Biophys. Biochem. Cytol. 8:467-482, 1960.

CHANDLER, R. L., and WILLIS, R.: An intranuclear fibrillar lattice in neurons. J. Cell Sci. 1:283-286, 1966.

GONATAS, N. K.: Subacute sclerosing leucoencephalitis: electron microscopic and cytochemical observations on a cerebral biopsy. J. Neuropath. Exp. Neurol. 25:177-201, 1966.

GONATAS, N. K., MARTIN, J., and EVANGELISTA, I.: The osmiophilic particles of astrocytes: viruses, lipid droplets or products of secretion? J. Neuropath. Exp. Neurol. 26:369-376, 1967.

HERNDON, R. M., and RUBINSTEIN, L. J.: Light and electron microscopy observations on the development of viral particles in the inclusions of Dawson's encephalitis (subacute sclerosing panencephalitis). Neurology 18 (Part 2):8-20, 1968.

HIRANO, A.: The fine structure of brain in edema. *In* Bourne, G. H. (Ed.): The Structure and Function of Nervous Tissue, Vol. II. New York, Academic, 1969, pp. 69-135.

HIRANO, A.: Neurofibrillary changes in conditions related to Alzheimer's disease. *In* Wolstenholme, G. E. W., and O'Connor, M. (Eds.): Ciba Foundation Symposium: Alzheimer's Disease and Related Conditions. London, Churchill, 1970, pp. 185-207.

HIRANO, A., and ZIMMERMAN, H. M.: Some effects of vinblastine implantation in the cerebral white matter. Lab. Invest. 23:358-367, 1970.

HIRANO, A., and ZIMMERMAN, H. M.: Glial filaments in the myelin sheath after vinblastine implantation. J. Neuropath. Exp. Neurol. 30:63-67, 1971.

HIRANO, A., ZIMMERMAN, H. M., and LEVINE, S.: The fine structure of cerebral fluid accumulation. X. A review of experimental edema in white matter. *In* Klatzo, I., and Seitelberger, F. (Eds.): Brain Edema. New York, Springer-Verlag, 1967, pp. 569-589.

JAKUS, M. A.: Studies on the cornea. II. The fine structure of Descemet's membrane. J. Biophys. Biochem. Cytol. 2(Suppl.):243-252, 1956.

KUNG, P. C., LEE, J. C., and BAKAY, L.: Vascular invasion by glioma cells in man: an electron microscopic study. J. Neurosurg. 31:339-345, 1969.

LEVENTHAL, H. R.. Electron microscopy of brain tumors. Clin. Neurosurg. 7:56-62, 1959.

LONG, D. M.: Capillary ultrastructure and the blood-brain barrier in human malignant brain tumors. J. Neurosurg. 32:127-144, 1970.

LUSE, S. A.: Electron microscopic studies of brain tumors. Neurology 19:881-905, 1960.

LUSE, S. A.: Ultrastructural characteristics of normal and neoplastic cells. *In* Homburger, F. (Ed.): Progress in Experimental Tumor Research. Philadelphia, Lippincott, 1961, pp. 1-35.

LUSE, S. A.: Electron microscopy of brain tumors. *In* Fields, W. S., and Sharkey, P.C. (Eds.): The Biology and Treatment of Intracranial Tumors. Springfield, Thomas, 1962, pp. 75-103.

Masurovsky, E., Benitez, H. H., Kim. S. U., and Murray, M. R.: Origin, development, and nature of intranuclear rodlets and associated bodies in chicken sympathetic neurons. J. Cell Biol. 44:72-191, 1970.

Perier, O., and Vanderhaeghen, J. J.: Subacute sclerosing leuco-encephalitis. Electron microscopic findings in two cases with inclusion bodies. Acta Neuropath. 8:362-380, 1967.

Peters, A., Palay, S. L., and Webster, H. deF.: The Fine Structure of the Nervous System. New York, Harper, 1970.

Popoff, N., and Stewart, S.: The fine structure of nuclear inclusions in the brain of experimental golden hamsters. J. Ultrastruct. Res. 23:347-361, 1968.

Raimondi, A. J.: Ultrastructure and the biology of human brain tumors. In Krayenbühl, H., Maspes, P.E., and Sweet, W. H. (Eds.): Progress in Neurological Surgery, Vol. 1. Chicago, Year Book, 1966, pp. 1-63.

Raimondi, A. J., Mullan, S., and Evans, J. P.: Human brain tumors: an electron microscopic study. J. Neurosurg. 19:731-759, 1962.

Ramsey, H. J.: Fibrous long-spacing collagen in tumors of the nervous system. J. Neuropath. Exp. Neurol. 24:40-48, 1965.

Sawada, T.: The fine structure of gliomas. Acta Med. Fukuoka 37:47-76, 1967.

Tani, E., and Ametani, T.: Intercellular contacts of human gliomas. In Zimmerman, H. M. (Ed.): Progress in Neuropathology, Vol. 1. New York, Grune & Stratton, 1971, pp. 218-231.

Zimmerman, H. M.: Some contributions of electron microscopy to problems in pathology. The Twenty-Fourth Middleton Goldsmith Lecture. Bull. N.Y. Acad. Med. 40:831-862, 1964.

Zülch, K. J., and Wechsler, W.: Pathology and classification of gliomas. In Krayenbühl, H., Maspes, P. E., and Sweet, W. H. (Eds.): Progress in Neurological Surgery, Vol. 2. Chicago, Year Book, 1968, pp. 1-84.

ZuRhein, G. M., and Chou, S. M.: Subacute sclerosing panencephalitis. Ultrastructural study of a brain biopsy. Neurology 18(Part 2):146-160, 1968.

ASTROCYTOMA

Duffell, D., Farber, L., Chou, S., Hartmann, J. F., and Nelson, E.: Electron microscopic observations on astrocytomas. Amer. J. Path. 43:539-545, 1963.

Luse, S. A.: Ultrastructure of reactive and neoplastic astrocytes. Lab. Invest. 17:401-417, 1958.

Luse, S. A.: Electron microscopy of normal optic nerve and optic nerve glioma. J. Neurosurg. 18:466-478, 1961.

Maxwell, D. S., and Kruger, L.: The fine structure of astrocytes in the cerebral cortex and their response to focal injury produced by heavy ionizing particles. J. Cell Biol. 25:141-157, 1965.

Mori, S., and Leblond, C. P.: Electron microscopic features and proliferation of astrocytes in the corpus callosum of the rat. J. Comp. Neurol. 137:197-226, 1969.

Smith, K. R., Schwartz, H. G., Luse, S. A., and Ogura, H. H.: Nasal glioma, a report of five cases with electron microscopy of one. J. Neurosurg. 20:968-982, 1963.

Tani, E., and Ametani, T.: Ciliated human astrocytoma cells. Acta Neuropath. 15:208-219, 1970.

CEREBELLAR SARCOMA

RAMSEY, H. J., and KERNOHAN, J. W.: Cerebellar sarcoma. J. Neuropath. Exp. Neurol. 23:706-718, 1964.

CRANIOPHARYNGIOMA

GHATAK, N. R., HIRANO, A., and ZIMMERMAN, H. M.: Ultrastructure of a craniopharyngioma. Cancer 27:1465-1475, 1971.

ZELICKSON, A. S.: Electron Microscopy of Skin and Mucous Membrane. Springfield, Thomas, 1963.

CRYPTOCOCCOSIS

COLLINS, D. N., OPPENHEIM, I. A., and EDWARDS, M. R.: Cryptococcosis associated with systemic lupus erythematosus. Light and electron microscopic observations on a morphologic variant. Arch. Path. 91:78-86, 1971.

EDWARDS, M. R., GORDON, M. A., LAPA, E. W., and GHIORSE, W. C.: Micromorphology of *Cryptococcus neoformans*. J. Bact. 94:766-777, 1967.

HIRANO, A., ZIMMERMAN, H. M., and LEVINE, S.: The fine structure of cerebral fluid accumulation. IV. On the nature and origin of extracellular fluids following cryptococcal polysaccharide implantation. Amer. J. Path. 45:195-207, 1964.

HIRANO, A., ZIMMERMAN, H. M., and LEVINE, S.: The fine structure of cerebral fluid accumulation: reactions of ependyma to implantation of cryptococcal polysaccharide. J. Path. Bact. 91:149-155, 1966.

HIRANO, A., ZIMMERMAN, H. M., and LEVINE, S.: The fine structure of cerebral fluid accumulation. VII. Reactions of astrocytes to cryptococcal polysaccharide implantation. J. Neuropath. Exp. Neurol. 24:386-397, 1965.

LEVINE, S., HIRANO, A., and ZIMMERMAN, H. M.: The reaction of the nervous system to cryptococcal infection — an experimental study with light and electron microscopy. *In* Zimmerman, H. M. (Ed.): Infections of the Nervous System: Proceedings of the Association for Research in Nervous and Mental Diseases. Baltimore, Williams & Wilkins, 1968, pp. 393-423.

TSUKAHARA, T.: Cytological structure of *Cryptococcus neoformans*. Jap. J. Microbiol. 7:53-60, 1963.

EPENDYMOMA

BRIGHTMAN, M. W., and PALAY, S. L.: The fine structure of ependyma in the brain of the rat. J. Cell Biol. 19:415-439, 1963.

ESCOLA PICO, J.: Die Feinstruktur versenkter Ependymzellen innerhalb von gliösen Narbenbereichen. Acta Neuropath. 3:137-143, 1963.

HIRANO, A., and ZIMMERMAN, H. M.: Some new cytological observations of the normal rat ependymal cell. Anat. Rec. 158:293-302, 1967.

MILHAUD, M., and PAPPAS, G. D.: Observations de cils dans les noyaux de l'habenula de chats adults. C. R. Acad. Sci. Paris 264:474-476, 1967.

MILLER, C. A., and TORACK, R. M.: Secretory ependymoma of the filum terminale. Acta Neuropath. 15:240-250, 1970.

RODRIGUEZ, E. M.: Ependymal specialization. III. Ultrastructural aspects of the basal secretion of the toad subcommissural organ. Z. Zellforsch. 111:32-50, 1970.

TENNYSON, V. M., and PAPPAS, G. D.: An electron microscope study of ependymal cells of the fetal, early postnatal and adult rabbit. Z. Zellforsch. 56:595-618, 1962.

WESTERGAARD. E.: The Lateral Cerebral Ventricles and the Ventricular Walls. I kommission hos Andelsbogtrykkeriet i Odense, 1970.

EPITHELIAL CYST OF SPINAL CORD

HIRANO, A., GHATAK, N. R., WISOFF, H.S., and ZIMMERMAN, H. M.: An epithelial cyst of the spinal cord. An electron microscopic study. Acta Neuropath. 18:214-223, 1971.

GIGANTOCELLULAR GLIOMA

LYNN, J. A., PANOPIO, I. T., MARTIN, J. H., SHAW, M. L., and RACE, G. J.: Ultrastructural evidence for astroglial histogenesis of the monstrocellular astrocytoma (so-called monstrocellular sarcoma of brain). Cancer 22:356-366, 1968.

HEMANGIOBLASTOMA

CANCILLA, P. A., and ZIMMERMAN, H. M.: The fine structure of a cerebellar hemangioblastoma. J. Neuropath. Exp. Neurol. 24:621-628, 1965.

RAMSEY, H. J.: Fine structure of hemangiopericytoma and hemangioendothelioma. Cancer 19:2005-2018, 1966.

MALIGNANT LYMPHOMAS

MALDONADO, J. E.: Ultrastructure of the myeloma cell. Cancer 19:1613-1627, 1966.

SORENSON, G. D., and THEILEN, G. H.: Electron microscopic observations of bovine lymphosarcoma. Ann. N. Y. Acad. Sci. 108:1231-1240, 1963.

TANI, E., AMETANI, T., KAWAMURA, Y., and HANDA, H.: Nuclear structures of primary malignant lymphoma in the brain. Cancer 24:617-624, 1969.

MEDULLOBLASTOMA

ISHIDA, Y., KAWAI, S., SATO, K., and NIIBE, H.: Electron microscopy of experimental cerebellar gliomas. Gunma J. Med. Sci. 13:79-90, 1964.

KADIN, M. E., RUBINSTEIN, L. J., and NELSON, J. S.: Neonatal cerebellar medulloblastoma originating from the fetal external granular layer. J. Neuropath. Exp. Neurol. 29:583-599, 1970.

MATAKAS, F., and CERVOS-NAVARRO, J.: The ultrastructure of medulloblastoma. Acta Neuropath. 16:271-284, 1970.

VOIGT, W. H.: Elektronmikroskipische Beobachtungen an menschlichen Medulloblastomen. Deutsch. Z. Nervenheilk. 192:290-309, 1968.

WAGA, S.: A histological and electron microscopic study on medulloblas-
tomas and cerebellar sarcomas. Arch. Jap. Chir. 34:436-454, 1965.

MENINGIOMA

CERVOS-NAVARRO, J.: Zur Feinstruktur endotheliomatöser Meningiome
des Menschen. Acta Neuropath. 8:141-148, 1967.
CERVOS-NAVARRO, J., and VASQUEZ, J.: Elektronenmikroskopische Untersuchungen über des Vorkommen von Cilien in Meningiomen. Virchow Arch. [Path. Anat.] 341:280-290, 1966.
CERVOS-NAVARRO, J., and VASQUEZ, J.: An electron microscopic study of
meningiomas. Acta Neuropath. 13:301-323, 1969.
GONATAS, N. K., and BESEN, M.: An electron microscopic study of three
human psammomatous meningiomas. J. Neuropath. Exp. Neurol.
22:263-273, 1963.
ISHIDA, Y., KAWAI, S., SATO, S., TAKAYANAGI, T., and KAWAFUCHI, J.: Electron microscopy of meningothelial meningioma. Gunma J. Med. Sci.
13:181-197, 1964.
KEPES, J.: Electron microscopic studies of meningiomas. Amer. J. Path.
39:499-510, 1961.
NAPOLITANO, L., KYLE, R., and FISHER, E. R.: Ultrastructure of meningiomas and the derivation and nature of their cellular component.
Cancer 17:233-241, 1964.
NYSTRÖM, S. H.: A study of supratentorial meningiomas. With special
reference to gross and fine structure. Acta Path. Microbial. Scand.
(Suppl.) 176:1-90, 1965.
ROBERTSON, D. M.: Electron microscopic studies of nuclear inclusions in
meningiomas. Amer. J. Path. 45:835-848, 1964.

NEURILEMOMA

CRAVIOTO, H., and LOCKWOOD, R.: Long-spacing fibrous collagen in
human acoustic nerve tumors. In vivo and in vitro observations.
J. Ultrastruct. Res. 24:70-85, 1968.
FISHER, E. R., and VUZEVSKI, V. D.: Cytogenesis of schwannoma (neurilemoma), neurofibroma, dermatofibroma, and dermatofibrosarcoma
as revealed by electron microscopy. J. Amer. Clin. Path. 49:141-154,
1968.
GIBSON, A. A. M., HENDRICK, E. B., and CONEN, P. D.: Intracerebral
schwannoma. J. Neurosurg. 24:552-557, 1966.
HARKIN, J. C.: Localization of the cellular site of collagen synthesis in
peripheral nerves by electron microscope autoradiography using
H3-proline. In Lüthy, F., and Bischoff, A. (Eds.): Proceedings of
the Fifth International Congress of Neuropathology. Amsterdam,
Excerpta Medica, 1966, pp. 861-863.
HARKIN, J. C., and REED, R. J.: Tumors of the Peripheral Nervous System.
Washington, Armed Forces Institute of Pathology, 1969.
PINEDA, A.: Submicroscopic structure of acoustic tumors. Neurology
14:171-184, 1964.
PINEDA, A.: Collagen formation by principal cells of acoustic tumors.
Neurology 15:536-547, 1965.
PINEDA, A.: The "lemmocyte" in peripheral-nerve tumors. J. Neurosurg.
22:594-601, 1965.

PINEDA, A.: Mast cells — their presence and ultrastructural characteristics in peripheral nerve tumors. Arch. Neurol. 13:372-382, 1965.

PINEDA, A.: Electron microscopy of the lemmocyte in peripheral nerve tumors (neurolemmomas). J. Neurosurg. 25:35-44, 1966.

RAIMONDI, A. J., and BECKMAN, F.: Perineurial fibroblastomas: their fine structure and biology. Acta Neuropath. 8:1-23, 1967.

RAMSEY, H.: Fibrous long-spacing collagen in tumors of the nervous system. J. Neuropath. Exp. Neurol. 24:40-48, 1965.

WAGGENER, J. D.: Ultrastructure of benign peripheral nerve sheath tumors. Cancer 19:699-709, 1966.

OLIGODENDROGLIOMA

GARCIA, J. H., and LEMMI, H.: Ultrastructure of oligodendroglioma of the spinal cord. Amer. J. Clin. Path. 54:757-765, 1970.

TANI, E., YAMASHITA, J., TAKEUCHI, J., and HANDA, H.: Polygonal crystal line structures and crystalline aggregates of cylindrical particles in human glioma. Acta Neuropath. 13:324-337, 1969.

VASQUEZ, J. J., and NAVARRO, J. C: Intranucleäre stabförmige Gebilde bei einem Oligodendrogliom. Acta Neuropath. 13:289-293, 1969.

PERINEURIUM

BURKEL, W. E.: The histological fine structure of perineurium. Anat. Rec. 158:177-190, 1967.

CRAVIOTO, H.: The perineurium as a diffusion barrier: ultrastructural correlates. Bull. Los Angeles Neurol. Soc. 31:196-208, 1966.

KRISTENSSON, K., and OLSSON, Y.: The perineurium as a diffusion barrier to protein tracers. Acta Neuropath. 17:127-138, 1971.

LIEBERMAN, A. R.: The connective tissue elements of the mammalian nodose ganglion. An electron microscope study. Z. Zellforsch. 89:95-111, 1968.

PILLAI, A. P.: A banded structure in the connective tissue of nerve. J. Ultrastruct. Res. 11:455-468, 1964.

RÖHLICH, P., and KNOPP, A.: Elektronenmikroskopische Untersuchungen an den Hüllen des *N. ischiadicus* der Ratte. Z. Zellforsch. 53:299-312, 1961.

WAGGENER, J. D., BUNN, S. M., and BEGGS, J.: The diffusion of ferritin within the peripheral nerve sheath: an electron microscopy study. J. Neuropath. Exp. Neurol. 24:430-443, 1965.

PITUITARY ADENOMAS

OLIVA, H., NAVARRO, V., and OBRADOR, S.: Microscopia electronica de los adenomas cromofobos de la hipofisis. Acta Neurochir. 14:141-153, 1966.

SCHELIN, U.: Chromophobe and acidophil adenomas of the human pituitary gland. A light and electron microscopic study. Acta Path. Microbiol. Scand. (Suppl.) 158:1-80, 1962.

ZANBRANO, D., AMEZUA, L., DICKMANN, G., and FRANKE, E.: Ultrastructure of human pituitary adenomata. Acta Neurochir. 18:78-94, 1968.

RENAL CLEAR CELL CARCINOMA

ERICSSON, J. L., SELJELID, R., and ORRENIUS, S.: Comparative light and electron microscopic observations of cytoplasmic matrix in renal carcinomas. Virchow Arch. [Path. Anat.] 341:204-223, 1966.

OBERLING, C., RIVIERE, M., and HAGUENAU, F.: Ultrastructure of the clear cells in renal carcinomas and its importance for the demonstration of their renal origin. Nature 186:402-403, 1960.

SELJELID, R., and ERICSSON, J. L.: Electron microscopic observations on specializations of the cell surface in renal clear cell carcinoma. Lab. Invest. 14:435-447, 1965.

ROSENTHAL FIBERS

HERNDON, R. M., RUBINSTEIN, L. J., FREEMAN, J. M., and MATHIESON, G.: Light and electron microscopic observations on Rosenthal fibers in Alexander's disease and in multiple sclerosis. J. Neuropath. Exp. Neurol. 29:524-551, 1970.

SCHLOTE, W.: Rosenthalsche "Fasern" und Spongioblasten im Zentral-nerven-system. I. Vorkommen in ventrikelfernen Reparationsgliosen; Darstellbarkeit der "Fasern" im Zellbild. Beitr. Path. Anat. 133:225-248, 1966.

SCHLOTE, W.: Rosenthalsche "Fasern" und Spongioblasten im Zentral-nervensystem. II. Elektronenmikroskopische Untersuchungen. Bedeutung der Rosenthalschen "Fasern." Beitr. Path. Anat. 133:461-480, 1966.

SCHLOTE, W.: Beitrag zum Vorkommen und zu Veränderungen der intra-cytoplasmatischen Filaments in Gliomen. Acta Neuropath. 8:108-112, 1967.

SCHOCHET, S. S., LAMPERT, P. W., and Earle, K. M.: Alexander's disease. A case report with electron microscopic observations. Neurology 18:543-549, 1968.

INDEX

All page numbers in *italics* refer to plates.